THE YOGA SUTRAS

OF PATANJALI

THE YOGA SUTRAS
OF PATANJALI

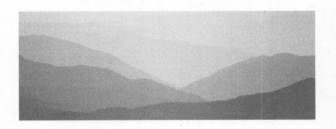

Translated and Introduced by
ALISTAIR SHEARER

❧ SACRED TEACHINGS

BELL TOWER ⚜ NEW YORK

Grateful acknowledgment is made to the following for previously
published material: *Faber and Faber Ltd., and Harcourt, Inc.:* Excerpt from
"Little Gidding" in FOUR QUARTETS, copyright 1942 by T. S. Eliot and
renewed 1970 by Esme Valerie Eliot, reprinted by permission of Faber
and Faber Ltd., and Harcourt, Inc.

Published by Bell Tower, New York, New York.
Member of the Crown Publishing Group.

Random House, Inc. New York, Toronto, London, Sydney, Auckland
www.randomhouse.com

Bell Tower and colophon are registered trademarks of Random House, Inc.

Originally published, in different form, by Wildwood House Limited,
London, under the title *Effortless Being: The Yoga Sutras of Patanjali,* in 1982.

Printed in the United States of America

DESIGN BY BARBARA STURMAN

Library of Congress Cataloging-in-Publication Data
Patañjali.
    [Yogasutra. English]
    The Yoga Sutras of Patanjali / translated and introduced by
Alistair Shearer.
        —(Sacred teachings)
    "Originally published in different form, by Wildwood House
Limited, London, under the title Effortless Being: the Yoga Sutras of
Patanjali, in 1982."
    1. Yoga—Early works to 1800. I. Shearer, Alistair. II. Series.
B132.Y6 P24313 2002
181'.452—dc21   2001024807

ISBN 0-609-60959-9

18

First American Edition 2002

CONTENTS

MY PRINCIPLE DEBT of thanks is to my teacher, Maharishi Mahesh Yogi, who has devoted his life to the revival of the wisdom of yoga. If there is anything worthwhile in my translation, it is solely due to what I have assimilated of his teaching.

Many other people have contributed to this project, through their advice, criticism, and enthusiasm. I'd like to thank especially: Frederick Smith, an accomplished Sanskritist who, en route from the University of Pennsylvania to Deccan College, Poona, drew my attention to many subtleties in the third and fourth chapters that I would otherwise have missed; Jack and Margaret Trevenna, who helped enormously in refining the final draft at a time when they themselves were under considerable pressure; and last, but by no means least, many thanks to Ruthie, who was so much help at the time, and whose company I still miss.

THE YOGA SUTRAS

OF PATANJALI

To MOST OF US suffering is a fact of life. It seems inevitable, despite all our attempts at consolation. The fundamental dissatisfaction of human beings has been the central concern of all religious and philosophical systems. Faced with our inability to remain happy, all the great teachers have adopted the most practical approach. The Buddha, for example, discouraged his followers from depending on anything external: leaders, dogmas, or unrealistic beliefs. Nor would he expound comforting metaphysical theories; he held that these were irrelevant. Instead, he presented his pupils with a straightforward and rational analysis of their predicament. He pointed out that all things are impermanent: that our lives are short, restricted, and, ultimately, unsatisfying. On its own this uncompromising diagnosis of the human condition would have been dismal indeed. Happily, the Buddha prescribed the cure. He called it "the path that leads to Enlightenment." It is a restatement of a perennial teaching that he had verified by his own experience.

This teaching is called yoga. According to yoga, we suffer because we live in ignorance. We are ignorant of our real nature. Our true nature lies beyond the restrictions of our careworn and humdrum existence, ecstatically free and untouched by suffering. Deep within the mind, beyond the faintest flicker of thought, it is experienced as an undying and omnipresent vastness. It is absolute consciousness. Animating everything in creation, this is the source and goal of all life. Yoga calls it the Self.

The nature of life is to grow toward an ever more perfect and joyous expression of itself. Each living being has a nervous system, no matter how rudimentary. This acts as a localized reflector of all-pervading consciousness, just as a mirror reflects light. The more developed the nervous system, the more it will express the qualities of pure consciousness—intelligence, creativity, and bliss. Yoga is the transformation into this Divine, and of this Divine into everything. Meditation is the key.

The whole thrust of evolution is to create increasingly complex systems that are capable of reflecting an ever greater degree of awareness. Science has realized that humans are more intelligent than animals because our neural organization is more evolved; as a result, we have more consciousness at our disposal. Yoga goes further. It says that the human nervous system is the crowning glory of creation, because it alone has the ability to reflect the unbounded source of life in its immaculate and radiant purity. Man is made in the image of God.

The desire to know the Self is implanted deep within each of us; a memory of Eden as old as the mind. However dimly perceived, this longing is the most refined expression of the dynamic urge to grow and progress that energizes all life and motivates every aspiration. Only when we realize our true nature, and the individual mind becomes infinite, shall we be satisfied. This Enlightenment is the first and last freedom; it is the state of effortless Being.

> We shall not cease from exploration
> And the end of all our exploring
> Will be to arrive where we started
> And know the place for the first time.
>   —T. S. ELIOT, "LITTLE GIDDING"

The quest for the Self has enthralled mankind since the dawning of desire. Ancient myths of every culture tell the same story of our search for wholeness. As the mind explores its own depths, it uncovers archetypal images that sustain and guide the journey inward. These are the signposts on the old road home, half-remembered from long ago. Each society hands down its stories of the great heroes who have made the journey before us as reminders and examples to those who follow. In Mesopotamia, the king of Erech, Gilgamesh, leaves his city and sets forth to find the plant of immortality "never-grow-old" that sprouts at the bottom of the Cosmic Sea. In ancient Greece, the nobly born Odysseus seeks his island home of Ithaca, while Jason sets sail on the search for the Golden Fleece. And in the very different setting of Arthurian England, the Knights of the Round Table ride out on that most sacred of missions, the quest for the Holy Grail.

Though the details of the myths differ with time and place, their pattern is the same. First comes the initial challenge, the call to a fuller life, the promise of a new state of being. If the hero has the courage to accept the challenge, with all its awesome implications of metamorphosis, he embarks on the crossing of the initiatory threshold that marks the beginning of the journey. This death and rebirth will have to be repeated many times before the quest is accomplished, for there are trials and dangers to be encountered on the way, and every transformation suffered is a dying to the old and a resurrection into the new. Such traveling requires fortitude and perseverance. The decisions to be taken are not easy—the unwary are soon tranquilized by triviality, the song of the sirens is alluring, and for every Galahad there are countless Launcelots.

But the deserving seekers are sustained by unseen help, those hidden agencies of fairy tale and legend. For the dedicated there will in time come the final achievement: the apotheosis. Now the traveler can return, transfigured, to live as an example and inspiration to all those yet to complete the quest.

These returned heroes are the great teachers, the seers, saints, and prophets, the spiritual leaders of mankind. Complete in themselves and reintegrated with the cosmos of which they are now a conscious instrument, they have reached the goal of yoga. With the seer of the *Taittirīya Upanishad,* their song rings out to all creation: "Oh wonderful! wonderful! wonderful!"

If any country has traditionally considered this quest to be the central purpose of human life, it is India. Her civilization has from earliest times been built on the bedrock of yoga. Yoga itself is not Indian, it is universal, but it is to that primeval land that we must look to trace the background of the *Yoga Sūtras.*

Our first glimpse of yoga on Indian soil is tantalizingly brief. It is the famous steatite seal excavated at Mohenjo-daro, in what is now Pakistan. Mohenjo-daro was one of the principal cities of the civilization that flourished in the Indus River valley nearly three thousand years before Christ. This was a vast and well-organized urban culture extending in a thousand-mile arc that stretched from the Indus across to Delhi and down to the coast of the Arabian Sea not far north of Bombay. It provides us with our earliest information of civilization in the Indian subcontinent.

The Indus Valley seal depicts a fertility god. He is wearing horns, like the figures discovered in the ruined citadels of Mesopotamia, has an erect phallus, and is surrounded by wild animals: an elephant, tiger, rhinoceros, and buffalo. In front of him sits a pair of deer. The figure is cross-legged in a yoga posture, on a low meditation couch like those still used by yogis in India today. He is the prototype of the later Hindu deity Shiva, "the auspicious one," also known as Pashupati, "the Lord of all creatures." The source of life and time, Shiva creates the universe through the rhythm of his eternal dance and presides over the processes of change and re-creation. He lives in the forests, the lord of yoga and protector of yogis, and as such he is worshipped as the "Conqueror of death" *(mrityum jaya)* and the "Giver of joy" *(shankara).*

This enigmatic seal, barely two inches square, is imprinted with the Indus Valley script that remains undeciphered to this day. It is one of the very few pieces of archaeological evidence that acts as a link between the great cultural unity that spanned the Indo-Mediterranean world in prehistoric times, and the first known Indian civilization that succeeded it. Like some mysterious cipher, encoded with the essential wisdom of yoga, the seal transmits a teaching that, since the dawn of history, has been inseparably linked with the primeval and regenerative forces that govern both man and beast.

The Indus Valley culture lasted until the middle of the second millennium B.C. No one knows for certain how or why it disappeared. All we do know is that contemporaneous with it thrived another, equally enigmatic culture, that of the Aryan people, who grouped themselves around the Saraswati river, now deep underground. Their sacred wisdom was encoded in the *Vedas,* which are mankind's oldest records of knowledge and the only surviving evidence of the Aryan civilization. They are richly poetic, sensuous descriptions of the eternal drama of the creation, maintenance, and dissolution of the universe, and are said to be truths intuited by enlightened seers *(rishis)* at the beginning of this cosmic cycle. They have been passed down orally through a hereditary succession of *pandits* to the present day. Although these recondite chants have remained virtually unfathomed by Western scholarship, they have been of immense importance in shaping the whole of subsequent Indian culture. In their written form they are the sacred books of Hinduism—that loosely related group of religious beliefs and practices that is the offspring of the Vedic and indigenous cultures. Indeed, they are still revered as the fount of all knowledge of orthodox Hindus, who regard them as the textbooks of eternal truth *(sanātana dharma)*.

Life in Vedic India revolved around the necessity of maintaining contact with the myriad celestial energies that uphold the universe. These are the *devas*—"the shining ones." This contact was essential to preserve the harmony of the cosmic hierarchy in which the human realm is only one among many. The way to sustain this universal order was twofold: through the performance of sacrificial ritual and the practice of yoga.

The *Vedas* reiterate that, if the cosmic order is

disrupted and the harmony between the various planes of creation broken, then suffering is the inevitable result. The Aryans saw no fundamental difference between the material and the spiritual worlds, or between the realms of mind and matter. Therefore it was of the utmost importance that thought, speech, and action be life-supporting— in harmony with all other levels of the universe. As they lived by a code that sought to embrace all aspects of life, their society was organized as a microcosm of the natural order. This was probably the origin of the later caste system. The specialized knowledge of sacrificial ritual was the province of the brahmins. Because of this tradition of priestly expertise, the brahmins have continued to command enormous respect among the orthodox up until modern times.

One group of Vedic texts, the *Upanishads,* is especially concerned with yoga. The oldest of the *Vedas* tells us that this knowledge is eternal and absolute, because it "dwells in the imperishable transcendental field of life" *(Rig Veda).*

In the forest hermitages of Vedic times, a group of pupils would gather around a teacher who instructed them in yoga and supervised their progress. We know that many such schools were still active at the time of the Buddha (around 600 B.C.), and that he studied with several teachers before his awakening. As a practical and nonritualistic way to expand awareness, yoga was considered a vital means of ensuring individual evolution. Whereas only the brahmins had access to the ritual procedures that maintained integration on a general level in society, yoga was open to all. It was the way for any individual, no matter what his social role, to purify his consciousness and live the full depth of life. The emphasis of yoga was, and still is, on the direct experience of the state of effortless Being. This wholeness transcends all the boundaries of the relative world, including those of social division.

The Buddha lived at a time when the Vedic rituals were no longer a unifying force in society. They had become a religion of outer trappings, mere ritualism and empty speculation. In the ruins of the Vedic civilization the first followers of the Buddha inaugurated the religion that was to irradiate almost all southeast Asia and the Far East.

There are many obvious similarities between this early Buddhism and the message of the *Yoga Sūtras*. The "noble eightfold path" closely resembles the "eight limbs of yoga," and the eight stages *(jhānas)* of Buddhist meditation are practically the same as the stages of *samādhi* delineated by Patanjali. Many of the crucial terms of the *sutras* are also found in the Buddhist canon: the causes of suffering *(kleshas)* are frequently referred to, as are the four virtues of friendliness *(maitri)*, compassion *(karunā)*, happiness *(mudita)*, and impartiality *(upekshāna)*. So are the adjective "unbounded" *(shūnya)* and the expression "the state of unclouded Truth" *(dharmameghasamādhi)*. Many other examples could be cited. Moreover, the whole atmosphere of Patanjali's *sutras* is one of an assured and tranquil lucidity reminiscent of the classical Buddhist scriptures.

Scholars have taken such parallels as proof that the *sutras* were heavily influenced by Buddhist teachings. It is more fruitful to see them as indications that both sets of texts drew on a common body of nonsectarian knowledge that had been available from time immemorial. Both were responses to the needs of the time, looking to a wisdom that is perennial.

It was this same wisdom which inspired a contemporary of the Buddha, Mahāvīra. He also turned to yoga, and applied its methodology to a dogmatic system that was austerely monastic and outside the tradition of Vedic orthodoxy. The result was Jainism.

In fact, each of the disparate elements of the Indian religious tradition are united by yoga; it is the hub around which they all revolve. The esoteric Tantric cults of Bengal adopted yoga as a means to ecstasy, and it was their baroque form of the teaching that was to provide techniques and ritual for the various sects, both Hindu and Buddhist, that flourished encapsulated in the remote Himalayan kingdoms.

But yoga is not confined to the esoteric. At the other end of the Indian religious spectrum lie the great epics, the *Mahābhārata* and the *Rāmāyana*. Finalized at the beginning of the Christian era, they originated much earlier. The epics are the lifeblood of popular religion in the subcontinent, and their stories are told, sung, danced, and acted by itinerant troupes who travel the length and breadth of the country even today. In many villages this is still the main form of education. A kaleidoscopic mixture of history, myth, and religious instruction, the epics proudly proclaim the exploits of the gods and heroes who practiced yoga and gloried in its power. The best known of these legends is the eighteenth chapter of the *Mahābhārata:* the *Bhagavad Gītā* or Song of God. In this the god Krishna, the embodiment of divine love, instructs Arjuna, who represents mankind, in the ancient teaching. Krishna emphasizes that yoga is essential to bring harmony and success to daily life.

He describes it as "skill in action," presenting it as a practical discipline, suitable for all people; a middle way that avoids the extravagances of asceticism on the one hand and sensuality on the other.

Similar in spirit to the teachings of Krishna were the movements of popular devotion that exploded on the Indian scene in the Middle Ages. It was the experience of the Divine, through yoga, that galvanized the poets, saints, and singers who dance their way so colorfully through the pages of medieval Indian history. Children in India are still traditionally brought up on the stories of these devotees of God who instituted both religious and social reforms—people like Rāmānanda in the south, Kabir the humble weaver from Benares, Chaitanya from Bengal, and Mīrabai, the beautiful Rajasthani princess.

This vein of joy has never been wholly lost, though it has often been obscured by lack of understanding. Even in recent years, it has sparkled through in such diverse personalities as Paramahansa Rāmakrishna, Ramana Maharshi of Tiruvannamalai, and the incomparable Bengali saint Ānandamāyī Mā. All these, and many more, celebrate in their own ways the blissful freedom of what Kabir once called "wandering in the ocean of deathless life."

> Nothing in all creation is so like God as silence.
> —MEISTER ECKHART

The word *yoga,* from the Sanskrit root YUJ, "to join," means "unity." Pānini, the grammarian who codified Sanskrit in the fourth century B.C. tells us: "That which unites is called *yoga.* He proceeds to define the word in three ways: "union" *(samyoga),* "coherence" *(sanyama),* and "the settling of the individual mind into its simplest and most expanded form of aware-ness" *(samādhi).* Thus it is synonymous with the original meaning of the word *religion*—from the Latin *religare,* "to bind back"—which is "reunification." Yoga is a way to restore our lost wholeness, our integrity as complete human beings, by unifying the personality around a center that is silent and unbounded.

Yet yoga itself is not a religion. It is undenomi-national, relying not on faith but on a number of techniques that gradually lead the individual to the direct experience of those truths on which religion rests. We can call it the inner spirit of religion, the colorless sap that nourishes and strengthens all parts of the tree of life impartially. When the knowledge of yoga is lost or distorted, the sap withdraws and the branches become brittle, wither, and eventually die. These are the times of spiritual drought, the dark nights of the soul when humanity is cut off from itself and the Divine. The *Purānas,* India's oldest sources of mythological lore, call them *kali yuga,* the times of blackness, when the goddess of destruction stalks the land, and ignorance and suffering prevail.

This is how the *Vishnu Purāna* describes these times of spiritual aridity:

> Society reaches a stage where property confers rank, wealth becomes the only source of virtue, passion the sole bond of union between husband and wife, falsehood the source of success in life, sex the only means of enjoyment, and outer trappings are mistaken for inner religion.

We live in such times today. Indeed, it would be hard to imagine a period in the history of the world that had greater need of the teachings of our text. Fortunately, it is a natural law that action provokes reaction. One reaction to the crisis of modern civilization is a tremendous growth of interest in the teachings of yoga over the past few years.

Yoga is relevant to our age because, far from being mystical or otherworldly, it is a teaching firmly grounded in physiological reality and can be understood in contemporary terms. We know that our experience of the world depends entirely on the state of our nervous system. This in turn is influenced by a host of factors—heredity, diet, environment, and so on. If the nervous system is fresh and rested, the body will be healthy and the mind alert and comprehensive. As a result, our thought will be powerful and clear and our actions, which are manifested thought, will be successful and rewarding. Conversely, if the system is tired, or strained, perhaps because of overactivity, or the influence of poor food, then our outlook will be restricted, the mind dull, and our actions ineffectual. Our life will become shallow and unsatisfying, a prey to all forms of negativity.

The techniques of yoga are methods of purifying the nervous system so that it can reflect a greater degree of consciousness and our lives can become an increasingly positive force in the world. If these techniques are correctly practiced, the whole nervous system is revitalized—the body enjoys better health and more energy, the rested mind is freed from the burden of past experience, and perception is restored to its primal freshness. Thought and activity become coherent and integrated, life becomes richer and more fulfilling.

Whether we choose to practice yoga, and interpret its benefits, within the framework of a conventional set of religious beliefs is up to us. Some people do, some don't. Yoga itself is neutral. It is a catalyst that allows us to grow in whichever direction is natural and life-supporting. Its methods work on the physical seat of consciousness, the nervous system, and, as far as yoga is concerned, a Hindu nervous system is no different from an Islamic or agnostic one. Each obeys the same laws that govern the operations of mind and body. Whoever practices yoga will be enlivened in his or her own way.

Every morning put your mind into your heart and stand in the presence of God all the day long.
—AN ANONYMOUS MONK OF THE
EASTERN ORTHODOX CHURCH

All the great religions have used the techniques of yoga to lead the mind inward to the silence that is the heart of the religious life. Each tradition has developed its own variations on the theme of our text. The dance and ritual movement of Islamic Sufism, the "Jesus prayer" practiced by the hesychast monks of Mount Athos, the martial art techniques of the Taoists in China—these are just some of the many ways of stilling the mind and reaching the silence within. Performed in the context of different faiths, they may differ in expression, but in essence they are one.

Such universality may seem strange to those brought up in the Judeo-Christian tradition. The hallmark of these religions is their emphasis on historical uniqueness, and by their own admission, they worship a jealous God. But even a cursory look at Christianity, for example, shows that its aims are perfectly compatible with the teachings of yoga.

The ultimate goal of the Christian life is union with God through loving contemplation. All the contemplative practices of the Catholic, Eastern Orthodox, and Protestant churches have their roots in the teachings of the desert fathers of Egypt and Syria. These doctrines were translated into Latin by John Cassian in the fifth century and are the starting point for all subsequent development of what Christianity calls "ascetic theology," the spiritual discipline of prayer and contemplation.

One of Cassian's chief authorities, the spiritual director Abbot Moses, explains:

> Our profession is the Kingdom of God, or the
> Kingdom of Heaven; but our immediate aim or

target is purity of heart, without which it is impossible
for anyone to reach that goal.

It is precisely this purity, in physical terms the result
of a pure nervous system, that is the "aim or target"
of yoga. To the yogi, no less than the Christian contemplative, purity is the handmaiden of the Divine.

Purity allows love, and love leads to devotion.
It is significant that the *Yoga Sūtras,* when referring
to the One as an object of devotion, use the word
īshvara. This comes from the root ĪSH, "to own" or
"to be able, powerful," and means "the Almighty,"
"the Lord." As such it has no sectarian connotations
whatever. Thus devotion can be directed toward
whatever aspect of the Divine we choose, and can
never become the monopoly of a particular cult or
creed. The teachings of yoga are "Beyond all divisions
of time and space." (3.54)

THE TEXT

The *Yoga Sūtras* are the most lucid and authoritative
of all the texts that serve as maps for the inner journey.
The result of many hundreds of years experience, the
sūtras are not necessarily the work of one author. They
were compiled by Patanjali, about whom we know
nothing except that he lived in India, probably in the

third century before Christ. Whatever their origin, the *sūtras* are the purest distillation of the knowledge of yoga. In just under two hundred crystalline verses, Patanjali codified a teaching of such translucence that he created one of the most remarkable works of spiritual literature in the world.

The word *sūtra* means "thread." As a literary style it is an aphorism of extreme brevity. All the Indian philosophical systems including the works on ritual, grammar, and meter, have used the *sūtra* form, as have many of the Buddhist writings. Because a *sūtra* is so succinct—Patanjali's average only six words each in the Sanskrit—a lively and varied tradition of commentary has arisen. Each new commentator brings the light of his own understanding to bear on the original gnomic texts; his conclusions then become part of the ongoing tradition.

The earliest commentary on the *Yoga Sūtras* dates from the fifth century, and is attributed to Vyāsa, of whom we know little. Tradition loosely identifies him with the compiler of the *Mahābhārata* and the *Purānas,* but *vyāsa* means "the arranger," and may well be a title given to renowned scholars rather than the name of an individual. Vyāsa's interpretation has been considered virtually indispensable for an understanding of the *sūtras,* and has been the starting point for nearly all subsequent commentary.

As the nodes of what was, and still is, essentially an oral teaching, the *sūtras* are almost like lecture notes, mnemonics. Each *sūtra* resembles a knot of the finest thread that must be teased out and unraveled, so that every inch of its meaning is displayed. Only then can the whole fabric of the teaching be woven together.

The spinning of this thread that guides us back out of the maze of ignorance is the work of a teacher *(guru)*. He, by definition, is one who enjoys the higher levels of consciousness described in the text. Teaching from his own experience, he is able to lead the pupil from darkness *(gu)* to light *(ru)*.

For those without such guidance, the structure of the *Yoga Sūtras* has caused much confusion. Because the text appears to be disjointed, modern scholars have set about dissecting it in an attempt to uncover the "original text" and identify later additions and influences. The consequences of such investigations is a tattered remnant composed of unrelated pieces. Each section is pronounced to be of a different age and origin and to represent a different view. As a result, the unity of the whole is destroyed and its practical value as a vital teaching is completely lost.

Orthodox Indian tradition has always treated its scriptures with profound respect. Throughout the ages the integrity of their content and the purity of their language have been zealously preserved. Sanskrit has remained almost unchanged since the fourth century B.C. and, as the vehicle of the sacred teachings, is itself considered divine. The word *samskrt* means "the perfected," and what is perfect is complete and beyond improvement. Given the innate conservatism of this tradition, it is extremely unlikely that the text of the *Yoga Sūtras* has altered significantly since it was compiled. Any innovative insight into its meaning will have taken the form of a fresh commentary, not an alteration of the text itself.

Over the centuries the *sūtras* have been thoroughly examined by some of the most acute minds in India. Early in the eleventh century the celebrated scholar al-Biruni made a translation into Arabic that exerted a seminal influence on Sufism. In practical terms, the *Yoga Sūtras* have remained a guiding light for generations of seekers after truth in both East and West, and are still considered the most authoritative source book on yoga today. Such continued esteem cannot be baseless.

Either we assume that Patanjali knowingly cobbled together a teaching that is inconsistent and in parts contradictory, or we accept that the text has an inner unity that has to be approached on its own terms. Our difficulty in understanding Patanjali's work as a unified whole lies not so much in the text itself as in our expectations of it.

The first thing to realize is that the *sūtras* are not intended to be only a literary work. Nor are they concerned with presenting a linear, sequential argument which is to be debated, and then accepted or refuted. Their purpose is to describe the stages of a journey that is unfamiliar to most of us. They view life from a vantage point that few of us realize exists.

Imagine a climber on the mountain slopes. He looks down on the villages with their cultivated fields spread out below. Another person, who has reached the summit, sends down a report that beyond these fields lie dense forests and then open plains, stretching to a vast and shoreless sea. The climber cannot share this experience, however much a description of it may excite his imagination.

Texts like the *Yoga Sūtras* are views from the mountaintop. Their purpose is to encourage and guide us, the climbers, to share their panoramic view. But the climb can only be accomplished in stages. Realizing this, teachers have often clothed their wisdom in parable, analogy, and provisional truth.

Patanjali's style, however, displays neither the charming blend of courtly and naturalistic imagery that characterizes the writings of the Taoists in China, nor the imaginative richness of Sufi poetry and fable. It is altogether more austere. Like some pure crystal, his message reveals its facets one by one. The whole picture is unfolded stage by stage and the teaching emerges gradually. In this way what is a complex and unfamiliar subject, the mechanics of consciousness, is broken down into easily manageable sections. Each section is self-sufficient, yet part of a greater whole.

It is particularly important that the truth be unfolded gradually when what is being conveyed is not knowledge in the normal sense but the transformation of consciousness itself. The teacher must apply *upāya*—"the skillful method"—he must teach on the level of the student's ability to understand. Otherwise his words may be recognized intellectually but their real meaning will not be grasped. Yoga confirms Blake's observation: "The fool sees not the same tree the wise man sees."

The Structure of the Text

The first four *sūtras* of Chapter 1 contain Patanjali's entire message in a nutshell: Yoga is the settling of the mind into silence, and only when the mind is silent can we realize our true nature, the effortless Being of the Self. The remaining one hundred and ninety *sūtras* are an expansion of this brief introductory statement.

It is common in Indian literature for the opening verses of a text to contain the whole subsequent teaching in seed form. This device of compaction is strange to us, who are more used to a linear argument gradually leading to a final conclusion. But it is perfectly logical. When we approach anything from a distance we see at first the whole, but only in its general outline. It is as we get closer that the component details become clear. The *Yoga Sūtras* begin by presenting us with a succinct overview of what is to follow, then, as our familiarity with the subject grows, the details are filled in, and their interlocking perspectives revealed.

Once the stage has been set, the first chapter proceeds by returning to the initial theme: the mind of the seeker. The fluctuations *(vrittis)* of the mind are defined (1.4–12) and then the stabilizing effect of yoga is presented as a counterbalance (1.13–16). What is yoga? Yoga is *samādhi* (1.17–18). The next ten *sūtras* (1.19–29) explain the prerequisites of *samādhi,* with particular attention to devotion as a means of approaching the Self. In this way some relationship is established between the seeker and the goal, which could otherwise remain too abstract and intangible. But the path is not always straightforward, and the *sūtras* continue by warning of the obstacles to be encountered (1.30–31), and the way to overcome them (1.32). From *sūtra* 33 to the end of the chapter we are presented with a more detailed expansion of the essential process, *samādhi*. *Sūtras* 33–40 deal with various ways of establishing the settled mind, and finally describe the actual mechanics of mental absorption *(samāpatti)* (1.41–47). Clear experience of the subtlest level of absorption brings us to *ritambharā,* the threshold of the unbounded. As this is a subject of considerable importance, it is picked up again and expanded in the third chapter. Chapter 1 ends by returning to the freedom described in the opening *sūtras,* now redefined as *nirbīja samādhi*— the unbounded consciousness of the Self.

This experience of the mind's dissolving into the Self is not the same as Enlightenment. Enlightenment is the state when this unbounded awareness is maintained at all times, during the states of waking, dreaming, and sleeping, no matter what the body and mind are doing. Just as it takes time for the mind to experience clearly the process of becoming boundless, it takes time to integrate this expansion into everyday life so that it is never lost. Enlightenment comes from the alternation of the completely settled mind and ordinary activity. In this way the Eternal gradually infuses the world of time.

Thus the second chapter, "Treading the Path," applies both to the realization of the state of unboundedness and to the stabilizing of this state in activity. As its title suggests, it describes all the stages of the journey until the goal is reached. Vyāsa begins his commentary on Chapter 2 with the words:

> The stage of yoga that is attained by the person with a calm mind has been explained. Now begins the explanation of how one with a restless mind can also attain yoga.

The chapter itself starts with the practical steps (sādhana), which must be taken by the aspirant, and continues by explaining the five causes of suffering (2.3). These are balanced by the remedy of the eight limbs of yoga (2.29). So the situation is presented from a different angle, and its solution explained in greater detail than previously. Where does suffering come from? We are told that it is the consequence of our past action, returned to us by the inevitable operations of the law of *karma* (2.12–14). As long as we are ignorant of our real nature, we shall continue to suffer.

Patanjali's examination of the eight limbs takes us to the end of the second chapter and into the third, which begins with a definition of what he calls the "heart of yoga," the delicate technique of *sanyama*. It is the practice of *sanyama* that results in the unfolding of the supernormal powers of the mind *(siddhis)*. These so-called miraculous powers include the ability to levitate, read the mind of another, and even become invisible. The entire chapter is taken up with a matter-of-fact enumeration of these extraordinary accomplishments, which are said to be the natural expression of the mind expanded by yoga. What is more, it is the technique of *sanyama* that actually develops the state of Enlightenment by training the mind to think on the very subtle level already delineated as *ritambharā* (1.48). The stages in the process of expansion are the "transformations" *(parināmas)* (3.9–12).

Chapters 2 and 3 can thus be seen to form one whole, which, broken in the middle to introduce *sanyama,* begins by analyzing the causes of suffering, continues by explaining the antidote, and triumphantly concludes with Self Realization.

The final chapter, having only thirty-four *sūtras,* is considerably shorter than its predecessors. It also appears somewhat piecemeal, and may possibly be incomplete. As it is, the chapter presents a number of scintillating ideas, flashes of philosophic lightning that dazzle us with their brilliance but vanish almost before we can examine what they reveal. Both mind and matter are said to contain their past and future states in an unmanifested form, and any change of state is an unfolding of latent potential. Thus, "our tendencies, which operate continuously to shape our lives" (4.9), are the results of our past actions; it is the cycle of cause and effect "maintained by the mind's bondage to its objects" that conditions all our thought and activity.

The way to destroy this "bondage" is to take the mind out of the realm of experience, the prison of time, causation, and space, allowing it to become unrestricted and universal. The more this universality is incorporated into the individual mind, the less that mind retains impressions of past actions. It will therefore be less ruled by desire. Most desires arise from a feeling of lack, but the mind that is infinite wants nothing. As the practice of yoga matures, desires cease to be the expression of need and become instead the spontaneous unfolding of love.

The second half of the chapter (17–34) deals with the relationship of the mind, intellect, and Self, and the process of "discrimination" *(viveka),* which leads to the highest *samādhi*—"the state of Unclouded Truth." The last six *sūtras* describe the final transformation into Enlightenment, the eternal freedom, in which "consciousness remains forever established in its own absolute nature" (4.34).

YOGA AS SUPREME KNOWLEDGE

The name of a philosopher, then, will be reserved for those whose affections are set, in every case, on the Reality.

—SOCRATES

In the ancient world, the philosopher was not merely a professional thinker, as he is today. Philosophy was considered a specialized study that led to a higher state of being. As such, it was directed toward a practical end, as was the study of music, dance, priestly ritual, and craftsmanship. Indian philosophy conducts an exhaustive study of the structure of the psyche and the range of its powers. It analyzes the senses and intellect, and studies the processes by which we experience the world. It also addresses itself to questions of ethics and morality. The primary concern, however, is not information but transformation. Philosophy is a means to Enlightenment.

The motto of the Indian philosopher was always: *"Ātmānam viddhi"*—"Know the Self." He was as closely allied to what we would call religion as his modern counterpart in the secular West is allied to the natural sciences. He shared the concerns of such early thinkers as Pythagoras, Plato, Plotinus, and, later, St. Augustine.

Such a man was expected to lead an exemplary life: a life of higher consciousness. The worth of his conclusions was judged by the extent to which his life mirrored his teachings. Plato demanded equally high standards from his Philosopher King: one who, living "in constant companionship with the divine order of the world, will reproduce that order in his soul, and, so far as man may, become godlike." In India, yoga was an indispensable part of the philosopher's training.

It is axiomatic in the yogic tradition that "knowledge is different in different states of consciousness" *(Rig Veda)*. In other words, our level of consciousness completely determines how much of the truth we see of any given situation. The clearer our minds, the more correctly we evaluate our experience. The state of Enlightenment is said to be complete knowledge, because it is based on the unchanging experience of the knower—the Self. Until this state is reached, any knowledge is ultimately baseless, because it depends only on the mind, which is a prey to passing moods and general instability. Patanjali categorizes everything that changes as "an object," in contradistinction to the one unchanging subject, transcendental consciousness. In one crucial sutra, breathtaking in its implications, he tells us that "The mind does not shine by its own light. It too is an object illumined by the Self" (4.19). Truth is that which does not change, and the unenlightened mind with its fluctuating opinions and ideas, is too partial and too unstable to be a reliable authority on ultimate matters. To believe that reality can be comprehended by the unenlightened intellect was, to the Indian philosopher, like "trying to catch the air with a pair of tongs" *(Maitrī Upanishad)*.

To satisfy the natural desire for truth, the Vedic seers formulated six approaches to the question of reality. These are called the *darshanas:* the six orthodox systems of Indian philosophy. Each system explores the object of study from a different angle, and true knowledge is considered to be the sum total of information provided by these systems. *Darshana* comes from DRSH, "to see," and means in this context "a point of view, a perspective." Each *darshana* has its own province and its particular job to do; each is complete in itself as far as it goes.

THE SIX SYSTEMS

1. *Nyāya,* a system of reasoning and logic that, employing dialectic, establishes the correct procedure for gaining knowledge of an object.
2. *Vaisheshika* identifies an object by those characteristics that differentiate it from any other.
3. *Sānkhya* then proceeds to enumerate all the various levels of the object, from its grossest, most surface level to its inner core. All these levels, and the timeless reality underlying them, can be directly experienced through yoga.
4. Yoga is the practical means of refining perception.
5. *Karma Mīmānsā* is the consideration of the entire field of action in order to determine which actions are most in accord with the force of evolution. It involves the study of the Vedic scriptures, which are guidelines for living. It also comprises the science of Vedic rituals, those technologies of the sacred which enliven the subtle energies of the universe and bring us into harmony with them. As a result, we enjoy their support in life.

6. *Vedānta,* the final *darshana,* is considered to be "the fulfillment of knowledge" (*veda:* "knowledge," *anta:* "end"). It synthesizes, then augments the knowledge of *Sānkhya* and Yoga by showing that ultimately any object is nothing but an expression of the infinite consciousness which is its essential nature.

Many people have been misled into thinking that these six systems are irreconcilable. This is because the conclusions of one may seem to contradict those of another. *Vaisheshika* makes no mention of God, whereas *Mīmānsā* is theistic; *Sānkhya* posits a cosmic duality of spirit and matter while *Vedānta* is uncompromisingly nondualist. But each system is merely a different, yet equally valid perspective on a many-sided reality. Each is a view from a different level of consciousness. Any apparent contradictions only serve to illustrate the limitations of one particular approach. Reality is too vast and wondrous to be contained within the boundaries of any mind-made system.

The *darshanas* function as a hierarchy that corresponds to a systematic growth of awareness. The first three relate to stages of understanding revealed by the exercise of the rational intellect of the waking state; in this they are recognizable in terms of con-

ventional Western philosophy. But the fourth *darshana,*
yoga, transforms the very nature and functioning of
waking-state awareness through exposing it to transcendental consciousness. This process throws a radi-
cally clearer light on reality. The last two *darshanas*
build on this new perspective and comprise increasingly subtle and holistic levels of perception and
illumination, far beyond any conventional rational
understanding.

ENLIGHTENMENT

In the growth to full Enlightenment, there are three
successive and distinct stages. The first stage is to
realize who and what we really are, for without self-
knowledge, how can we hope to understand the
outside world and all that lies beyond our little self?
True self-knowledge is to have the immortal, transper-
sonal Self permanently established in our awareness.
Then the surface of our life, our individual mind, is
united to its base, the cosmic Self, which is experienced as an unbroken substratum of subjective awareness—"I AM." No matter what else is happening in
our experience, the Self is there as an undisturbed witness. When this level is clearly experienced in deepest meditation, there is what is called Self-realization;

when it is lived continuously through the transient states of waking, dreaming, and deep sleep, there is the first stage of Enlightenment, technically known as Cosmic Consciousness *(turīyatīt chetanā).*

The characteristic of Cosmic Consciousness is that there is a separation experienced between the inner, spiritual reality of the Self—silent, unmoving, and utterly stable—and the ever-changing activity of the outside world. Cosmic Consciousness is described in the literature of yoga as *jīvanmukti* ("liberation in life"). Its structure is explained by *Sānkhya* and achieved through the practical teachings and techniques of yoga. The *Yoga Sūtras* is the principal manual and teaching text of this essential stage of Enlightenment. The experience of Cosmic Consciousness is the source of many dualistic teachings in the great spiritual traditions, those confessions that emphasize the separation of spirit and matter and extol the majesty of inner freedom over and above the unsatisfactory nature of the outside world. For *jīvanmukti* is indeed eternal freedom, but it is freedom on the basis of a radical duality—Self and other—it is not yet the glory of full Enlightenment.

The second phase, which begins to resolve this existential duality, is the state when the infinity of the subjective Self begins to be infused into the objective, relative world, illuminating it in the celestial light of the Divine. This stage, the experience of which has given rise to the theistic, devotional teachings in the great traditions, is technically known as God Consciousness *(bhagavad chetanā)* and is explained in detail by the *darshana* of *Karma Mīmānsā*. Its principal explanatory text is the *Karma Mīmānsā Sūtras*.

The third and final stage, the full maturing of Enlightenment, is when the unbounded Self overflows, as it were, into the bounded world of time and space, and everything—all objects, all experience— is perceived as nothing less than the unbinding and temporary modification of that one infinite Radiance which is my Self. All previously held opposites are transcended: The relative is the form of the formless Absolute, the limited world of matter is but the expression of the infinite Spirit, and Eternity is lived through all the passing phases of time. It is this exalted state of Unity the *Bhagavad Gītā* lauds when it describes the accomplished yogi as:

> He whose self is established in yoga, whose vision everywhere is even, sees the Self in all beings and all beings in the Self.

> —CHAPTER 6, VERSE 29

Years later, Blake poetically described his own experience of Unity as being spontaneously able

> To see a world in a grain of sand
> And a heaven in a wild flower,
> Hold infinity in the palm of your hand
> And eternity in an hour.

Unity Consciousness *(brāhmī chetanā)* is the highest state, the pinnacle of evolution, when the individual lives in, and as, the very Divine. It has been celebrated in the nondual teachings of all the great traditions, and in the Indian context is the province of *Advaita Vedānta,* whose unified perspective enfolds and completes all the other, more provisional and partial *darshanas.* The seminal text is the *Vedānta* (or *Brāhma*) *Sūtras.*

Each sacred tradition encompasses different philosophical or spiritual viewpoints that vary according to the level of Enlightenment that has been reached. In orthodox Islam, for example, the separation of the transcendent Allāh from His creation is unremitting, and to deny this separation is to risk blasphemy. It took the esoteric contemplative schools of Sufism often persecuted by uncomprehending orthodoxy, to mature this partial perspective into one of Union with Beloved, an ecstatic unity that is celebrated in poetry, dance, and architecture. And in Buddhism, the early, or *Theravāda* schools, whose understanding was based on their experience of Cosmic Consciousness, tended to advocate an austerely circumscribed life predicated on a reclusive transcendence of the material world as a strategy to develop the first stage of enlightenment. Later, many of the *Mahāyāna* schools —active today mainly in their Tibetan (*Dzogchen* and *Mahāmudrā*) and Japanese (Zen) forms—were inspired by their experience of Unity Consciousness to develop the life-negating philosophies of the *Theravāda* into all-inclusive, life-affirming, and compassionate teachings that sought to bring all sentient beings to full enlightenment.

Sānkya and Yoga

The intellectual understanding of the experiences gained through yoga is provided by the *Sānkhya* system. This divides the cosmos into two complementary principles: *purusha* and *prakriti*. *Purusha* is the subjective aspect of life, the essence of mind that Patanjali calls "the Self." *Prakriti* is the primal substance, the matrix of all life, the matter-energy out of which arises the whole objective creation that the *sūtras* call "the world." The world is a manifestation of the Self, although paradoxically the two are, in fact, eternally distinct. *Prakriti* depends on *purusha* for her life, as the earth depends on the sun, yet *purusha* remains ever unaffected by the activities of his consort. *Sānkhya*—the word means "enumeration"—categorizes the hierarchy of principles that proceed from the effects of *purusha* within *prakriti*. *Prakriti* is composed of three constituent energies: the *gunas*. These are:

1. *Rajas,* the creative energy.
2. *Tamas,* the retarding and moderating energy that checks the activity of *rajas.*
3. *Sattva,* the harmonizing energy that integrates *rajas* and *tamas.*

Everything in creation is composed of a combination of these three energies. Before creation the *gunas* are perfectly balanced, but when this equilibrium is disturbed the universe begins to manifest, and the entire world of name and form arises in all its variety. Manifestation proceeds through a series of increasing gross levels *(tattvas)* that together constitute the objective world.

The whole purpose of the manifestation of these *gunas* from their state of equilibrium in the undisturbed *prakriti* is to bring about a state in which their eternal separateness from the Self is realized. When this is achieved the Self is liberated from "the world" and endures as a joyful and silent witness of all activity, including that of the body and mind. This is the state of freedom, when we realize that our real nature is, and always has been, the immortal and unattached spirit that animates all manifestation.

We are used to thinking of the mind as belonging to the subjective side of life. *Sānkhya,* however, disagrees. It classifies the mind as part of objective *prakriti,* and concludes that it is external to us, because we are the Self. *Sānkhya* is very precise in its delineation of the different parts of what we loosely call "mind." It divides the individual consciousness into three distinct components and calls them: mind *(manas),* intellect *(buddhi),* and ego *(asmitā).*

Manas, from the root MAN, "to think," is that part of the individual consciousness that thinks and feels.

Buddhi comes from BUDH, which means "to decide" or "to discriminate." The intellect is the faculty of choice. It is the quiet phase of our inner life that appraises, and discriminates between, the thoughts entertained by *manas.* As such it is crucial in life, for we are free to choose how we act and who we are. It is the intellect that determines our sense of identity.

According to *Sānkhya,* we mistakenly consider the intellect to be the source of consciousness within us.

It is this error that gives rise to the individual ego-sense *(asmitā),* which means "I-AM-ness." We think "I am happy," "I am sad," "I am doing such and such." This feeling of limited individuality is the critical delusion that is ultimately responsible for all the suffering and folly of human life. To identify completely with the individual ego is "ignorance of our real nature" because the ego is no more than a contraction of the all-pervading Being that is our essence. We sell our birthright for a mess of pottage.

How does this disastrous ignorance come about?

Imagine a glass of water standing on a sunlit table. The water is colored green, and the sun streams through it, casting a green glow across the table. Because the glow is green, and there is no green light coming through the window from outside, one might think that the glass was the source of light. But if the water were gradually purified, so that the dye was weakened little by little, not only would the sunlight filtering through the water become increasingly bright and clear, but it would be ever more apparent that the source of light was in fact not the glass but the sun.

Because the intellect is clouded and dull (the green color in our analogy), it considers itself to be the source of consciousness. But in truth, the individual intellect is merely the result of infinite consciousness being reflected through a particular nervous system. Failure to realize this produces egoism, the limited sense of "self" (2.6). But if the intellect is gradually purified by yoga, it eventually becomes able to discriminate between itself and the unlimited consciousness it reflects. The petty limitations of egoism are transcended, one consequence of which is that we no longer make the mistake of seeking security outside ourselves.

Like everything else, the intellect is a compound of the three *gunas*. Yoga is concerned with purifying the density of these *gunas* as they operate in the intellect so that the ability to discriminate is no longer obscured. Yoga first removes the dullness of *tamas,* then the agitation of *rajas,* finally revealing the intellect in its *sattvic* purity, transparent to the Self. This is supreme knowledge. "One who has attained complete discrimination between the subtlest level of mind and the Self, has no higher knowledge to acquire" (4.29).

We have seen how *Sānkhya* presents the hierarchy of creation arising from the pure consciousness of the Self. Grosser than the Self is individual ego that experiences, intellect that decides, and mind that feels and thinks. Grosser still are the senses. But there is

still the outside world to consider; life does not stop
with the senses. *Sānkhya* concludes its enumeration of
the different levels of manifestation by locating three
more *tattvas:* the *karmendriyas, tanmātras,* and *mahābhūtas.*

The *karmendriyas* are the faculties of action: speech,
grasping, walking, evacuating, and procreating. These
work with the senses in order to connect the mind
with the manifest world of objects. Whereas the
senses are passive, receptive, the faculties of action
are dynamic. The *tanmātras* are the essences of the
objects of the five senses of perception. They are:
sound, the essence of all we hear; texture, the essence
of all we touch; form, the essence of all we see;
flavor, the essence of all we taste; and odor, the
essence of all we smell. Lastly, as the grossest level
of manifestation, the *mahābhūtas,* are the five physical
elements out of which the entire material universe
is created. These are *ākāsha* (the subtle space that
interpenetrates all matter), air, fire, water, and earth.
Each respective element signifies a particular quality
of existence: connectedness, volatility, dynamism,
adaptability, and stability.

Because the senses exist primarily to present the
mind with experience of the outside world, their
ability to fulfill the mind's longing for truth is limited.
The range of sensory experience is confined to those

aspects of creation arising from the five elements. But the Self lies far beyond the relative, finite world, and just beyond the intellect. This is why it can never be experienced by the senses but can only be appreciated by the purified intellect *(buddhi sattva)*.

Each level in this hierarchy is linked. Thus each *tanmātra,* already associated with a particular sense, expresses itself in one of the five elements. Thus there is an intimate connection between hearing sound and its medium *ākāsha.* Similarly, touch is linked with texture and air, sight with form and fire, taste with flavor and water, and smell with odor and earth. The importance of these correspondences between the various levels of life is that a mind operating from the subtlest level, the innermost realm of *purusha,* can influence any relatively grosser level of creation it wishes. This is just like a gardener's ability to influence the whole plant by simply watering its roots. This skill is the basis of the "supernormal powers" described in Chapter 3.

The Eight Limbs

In Chapter 2 we are given a succinct summary of Patanjali's teaching in what he calls "the eight limbs of yoga" *(ashtavangani).* These eight interrelated parts cover all the areas of an individual's life. They are:

1. The Laws of Life *(yama):*
   nonviolence *(ahimsā)*
   truthfulness *(satya)*
   integrity *(asteya)*
   chastity *(brahmacharya)*
   nonattachment *(aparigraha)*
2. The Rules for Living *(niyama):*
   simplicity *(shaucha)*
   contentment *(santosha)*
   purification *(tapas)*
   refinement *(svādhyāya)*
   surrender to the Lord *(īshvarapranidhāna)*
3. Posture *(āsana)*
4. Breathing exercises *(prānāyāma)*
5. Retirement of the senses *(pratyāhāra)*
6. Focusing of attention *(dhāranā)*
7. Meditation *(dhyāna)*
8. The settled mind *(samādhi)*

Many commentators have assumed that the eight limbs are sequential stages on the path of yoga. They have seen the first two limbs, *yama* and *niyama,* essentially as prerequisites for the following six, and concluded that the final stage, *samādhi,* is only reached after years spent perfecting the preceding stages. This is only half the picture. It is true that the sequence of *āsanas, prānāyāma,* and meditation comprise any daily routine of yoga. It is also true that total *samādhi* is the result of the other seven limbs being fully developed. But the word *samādhi* is a general one, meaning "the settled *(samā)* mind or intellect *(dhi)*." As we have seen, there are different levels of *samādhi (samprajnata, nirbīja*—1.17; 1.51; etc.), and the experience of complete unboundedness is only the most refined of a number of levels of tranquillity. It is the settling down of the mind, to whatever degree, that right from the beginning of the path is responsible for perfecting and coordinating all the other limbs. Even the more shallow stages of *samādhi* enjoyed to begin with bring very deep rest to the entire system. The reduced metabolic rate enables accumulated stress and tension to be neutralized. While the body experiences this profound rest the mind is bathed in silence. Familiarity with this rested state will result in a healthier nervous system; a calmer, clearer mind; and a more harmonious and responsible way of living. These, in turn, are conducive to *samādhi,* and so the whole process is cumulative. Regular meditation leads to greater depths of inner silence, until eventually the system is pure enough to experience the total restfulness of the Self, that immensity in which "all activity has ceased" (1.51).

It is significant that Patanjali uses the word "limb" *(anga)*. The eight limbs of yoga together constitute one body and, as in any body, each limb grows simultaneously, in proportion to all the others, until full development is reached. It is an organic process. Had Patanjali wished to emphasize the idea of sequential steps, each to be completed before the next begins, he would have used a word such as *bhumi,* which signifies a stage in yoga. As it is, his message is clear. Each limb is joined to the others, balancing and strengthening them, as an integral part of a greater whole.

The body of yoga grows by itself, spontaneously. No amount of conscious effort to practice nonviolence, simplicity, integrity, and so on will achieve the desired effect. Any attempt to imitate what is considered a higher state can only result in strain, and is a contradiction in terms, like trying to relax. These qualities blossom naturally, as a result of right meditation. Real change comes from within, for "any change into a new state of being is the result of the fullness of nature unfolding inherent potential" (4.2).

A similar confusion has arisen over what are considered to be the four separate kinds of yoga: *hatha*—the yoga of the body; *jnana*—the yoga of the mind; *bhakti*—the yoga of devotion; and *karma*—the yoga of action. These are held to be appropriate to the four basic types of human personality: physical, intellectual, emotional, and practical. As such, they are believed to be mutually exclusive paths to Enlightenment. While it is true that these are valid archetypes, it would be truer to say that the four divisions are the interrelated areas of life, different but complementary.

This is why they are all included in Patanjali's teaching. Yoga strengthens each area simultaneously, for it is a holistic discipline that aims to balance and harmonize the various aspects of the individual personality, not to encourage any existing imbalance. Its goal is a state of completeness in which the body, mind, and heart are fully coordinated, and as a result all activity becomes as effortless as ripe fruit dropping off a tree.

It is impossible to convey the exact meaning of the eight "limbs" in translation. Sanskrit is a language of such compression that one word may carry many nuances of meaning for which we have no succinct equivalent. Some expansion is necessary:

Yama the first limb, sums up the qualities displayed by the sages. It also describes the inherent characteristics of life as seen by the wisdom eye of Enlightenment.

Ahiṃsā, to us the concept of "nonviolence" may have a limited connotation, political or pacifist, but the Sanskrit denotes a dynamic peacefulness that is prepared to meet all situations with a loving openness. It is the state of living free from fear.

Satya means impeccability in thought, speech, and action.

Asteya means "not stealing," in the wide sense of not laying claim to anything that is not really ours. There are many levels of misappropriation, but all are the expression of a feeling of lack. We "steal" as long as we identify with the limited self, the ego, and are ignorant of our real nature, which is a fullness of Being that needs no addition.

Brahmacharya means literally "moving in the Immensity" or "living in Reality," but from earliest times it has been understood to refer to the sublimation of the life force that is normally expressed as sexuality. Thus *brahmacharya* has frequently been translated as "celibacy," by which sexual continence is meant.

This has led to much confusion. True yoga is a natural process, and has no place for repression, whether of the ego, sex, or anything else. Such an attitude of forced control is against life, and can only result in strain and tension incurred in the name of some supposedly "higher" ideal. However, as we progress on the path of yoga, needs and desires become more refined. Sexuality is one area of experience that typically tends to aberration, becoming narrowly confined to the habitual need for release of tension and dissatisfaction, rather than the magnification of an already existing happiness. Nourished by yoga, a wider loving-awareness that is present at all times begins to develop. Such all-inclusiveness is the natural state of awareness; it has its own economy, self-sufficient and unforced. And if such a transformation is experienced, it will only be because the limited self, which is always more or less motivated by the need to overcome its chronic and anxious sense of separation through repetitive and unexamined behavior patterns, has been transcended. Transcendence has nothing to do with suppression, and *brahmacharya* does not mean "self-control" as normally understood. It is a state of self-sufficient wholeness, an innocence that is its own ecstasy.

Promiscuity—the word actually means "lack of discrimination"—in many areas of life is a way in which vital energy is often dissipated. Thinking and talking, as much as acting, are expressions of a power that increases if it is used wisely, and diminishes if it is not. *Brahmacharya* should be taken, in its widest sense, as true "chastity."

Aparigraha, literally "not grasping," has often been interpreted to mean assuming an attitude of renunciation, or cultivating a mood of being unattached to "worldly things." In fact, *aparigraha* refers to the state that comes spontaneously as the mind begins to experience the effortless Being of the Self. When the awareness starts to expand, it is able to view the world in a more generous perspective. As the practice of yoga advances, the individual derives his or her sense of identity less and less from self-images that must be compulsively adhered to, and more and more from a feeling of flexible and disinterested universality. The wise live naturally in the state of nonattachment; they are in the world but not of it.

The Rules for Living *(niyama)* constitute the second limb. Whereas *yama* refers to principles that, whether we realize it or not, uphold the very nature of life, *niyama* applies these general principles to the individual's life, discussing the qualities that grow with the practice of yoga.

Shaucha is usually translated as "cleanliness." While cleanliness is of course aesthetically desirable and necessary to maintain the optimum functioning of the nervous system, the word also describes a mind which is clear, uncluttered, and straightforward. Such clarity comes from *samādhi,* which is awareness at its most simple and unsullied. *Shaucha* is that purity the Bible calls being "poor in spirit."

Santosha: contentment, satisfaction. The equanimity that sees things as they are, undistorted by expectation, need, or fear.

Tapas has several related meanings: "fire," "heat," "brilliance," "ardor." It is usually translated as "austerity," and as a result the popular image of yoga is of a discipline involving asceticism or mortification. In fact, the word describes yoga as a process of transmutation, an inner alchemy that burns away the dross of imperfection. This purification is as much physical as moral or intellectual. As we have seen, meditation provides the nervous system with such deep rest that the negative effects of past experience—the stress caused by fatigue, repressed emotion, anxiety, and so on—are dissolved. This purification is natural, because it is the nature of the body to throw off any impurities. Nevertheless, in extreme cases the release of stress can take bizarre forms, and many of the fantastic and occult experiences loosely called "spiritual" are in fact nothing more than perceptual or emotional distortions caused by purification. The path is long and much has to be learned on the way. One common effect of purification is the experience of bodily heat. This may be concentrated at the subtle energy centers *(chakras),* or spread over the abdomen or chest, or along the spine. In the devotional context of Christian mysticism, this phenomenon is known as "the fire of love" *(incendium amoris).* Purification, the "resurrection of the body," is the very essence of yoga; it is facilitated by the treatments of Ayurveda, the indigenous Vedic system of natural medicine.

Svādhyāya means "study conducive to self-knowledge," and refers specifically to study of the scriptures. These records are spiritual "food," nourishing the personality and imbuing the mind with positive and elevating influence. They also serve as a practical guide by explaining experiences that are encountered by the yogi. In a more general sense, *svādhyāya* refers to the refined perception that comes from purification.

Īshvarapranidhāna is a compound of *īshvara* "Lord," and *pranidhāna* "devotion, surrender, application." Technically, *īshvara* is the name given to the very subtlest level of relative creation. This is the realm of the personal God, the creator, as distinct from the impersonal Godhead. Devotion is a means of cultivating the finer levels of feeling, without which no real progress on the spiritual path is possible. It may be directed in various ways—to one's concept of God, a teacher, a loving partner, or humanity in general— depending on the context in which it arises. The end result, the awakening of the finest levels of feeling, will eventually lead the devotee to appreciate the subtlest level of life.

The third limb is *āsana,* the physical postures that strengthen. These are physical exercises that strengthen and rejuvenate the body, releasing chronic muscular tension and freeing energy blocked at points of stress in the system. There are over eighty of these postures: "the lotus," "the fish," "the cobra," "the peacock," "the tree," and so on. Such organic names emphasize the naturalness of the discipline; they also suggest the yogi's unity with all life. We are told the postures should be "comfortable" (2.46) and that they are "mastered when all effort has been relaxed" (2.47). They also suggest the yogi's unity with all life.

Next come the breathing exercises *(prānāyāma).* The Sanskrit is usually taken to mean control *(yama)* of the breath *(prāna).* Actually, this is a misunderstanding. If we parse *prānāyāma* correctly, we get *prāna* and *ayāma* (the short last "a" of *prāna* and the short first "a" of *ayāma* elide by the rules of Sanskrit grammar to form one long *ā*). Strictly speaking, *prāna*—cognate with the Greek *pneuma* and the Chinese *chi*—does not just mean "breath" but the cosmic life-energy that manifests on the gross level as breath in living creatures. *Ayāma* means "expansion, increase." Thus, *prānāyāma* comes to mean "expansion and increase of the life-energy." In other words, it is the process whereby the ordinary and relatively weak manifestation of *prāna* in the nervous system is purified and strengthened. Breathing exercises form part of this process, allowing the refined *prāna* to penetrate deeper into the nerves *(nādis)* of both gross and subtle anatomies and release blocks of accumulated stress, which in yogic terms is the whole content of held and unresolved past experience—trapped memories, emotions, desires. As the nervous system becomes pure, this vitalizing flow of energy in the gross and subtle bodies increases. The resultant purification can be dramatic, often passing for genuine "spiritual" experience. In the yogic tradition, such symptoms have been minutely documented in the teachings of *Kundalinī Yoga,* whereas in the framework of Christianity, understood as the workings of the Holy Spirit, this purifying readjustment of the system gave rise to such Pentecostal events as speaking in tongues, and the physical movements that inspired such eponymous sects as the Quakers and the Shakers.

Breath and thought are two complementary expressions of *prāna;* they go together. When the breathing is calm, the mind automatically becomes more settled. One of the meanings of *nirvāna* is "without breath."

These postures and breathing exercises are together commonly known as *Hatha Yoga.* The most familiar aspect of yoga in the West, *Hatha Yoga,* is far more than a system of mildly esoteric keep-fit exercises. Its concern is to purify the gross and subtle levels of the nervous system so they can support the finer neuro-logical activity that is the physical basis for higher states of consciousness. *Hatha Yoga* is a preparation for the heart of yoga: meditation. This heart is also known as *Rāja Yoga,* the Royal Way. One of the oldest and most authoritative *Hatha Yoga* texts, the *Goraksha Samhitā,* clarifies the relationship between *hatha* and *rāja:*

> The scientific teaching of *Hatha Yoga* is like a ladder. Those who wish to reach the higher realms of the Royal Way climb up it.

The fifth limb is retirement of the senses *(pratyā-hāra).* As the mind begins to settle, the attention moves inward, no longer distracted by the outside world. "The senses retire from their objects, by following the natural inward movement of the mind" (2.54). The mind is always drawn to something that will give it greater satisfaction; it is like a bee that, seeking nectar, moves from one flower to the next. Because of this movement it is often thought that the mind must be restrained if it is to settle into quietness. In fact, the art of yoga is to allow the natural impetus of the mind to lead it inward to its own source, for it is this unbounded area that is the most satisfying thing in life. Once pointed in the right direction, the mind will begin to settle down of its own accord. It needs no control or forcible restraint.

Pratyāhāra can be translated as "in the direction of food." Like the mind, the senses are charmed by whatever they find most pleasing. It is precisely this orientation that leads them to follow the mind inward in meditation. There is no suggestion here of abstinence from sensory pleasures. On the contrary, the more the senses are refined, the greater the riches they reveal. *Pratyāhāra* is the cleansing of the doors of perception.

Having discussed yoga in terms of the world, the body, and the senses, Patanjali proceeds to the mind. He calls the realm of the mind "the heart of yoga, more intimate than the preceding limbs." This "heart" is threefold:

Dhāranā—steadiness of mind. *Dhāranā* means "holding," and describes the focusing of attention on an object. This is not the same as concentration, which in its modern usage implies a sustained effort, but a directed type of awareness. When perfected, this steadiness is called "one-pointedness" *(ekāgratā)*. The longer the mind can remain effortlessly focused, the more powerful it becomes.

Dhyāna—meditation. This is the process of the mind's activity becoming increasingly refined and more subtle while a thread of awareness is spontaneously maintained.

Samādhi—the settled mind—is the most delicate state of awareness.

Indeed, I tell you truly, any object you have on your mind, however good, will be a barrier between you and the inmost truth.

—MEISTER ECKHART

The heart of yoga is the practice of settling the mind into a state of absolute stillness. To accomplish this the normal mechanics of perception are used, but in an inward direction.

Our attention is usually directed outward. The

mind is focused, through the senses, on some object. At this moment your attention is focused through your eyes on these words. Later, you may turn on the radio and your attention will then focus through your ears. We know that there are levels of an object that are too subtle for our senses to experience unaided. Some things can only be seen through a microscope; we can hear some sounds only through an amplifier. Our perception is normally limited to the gross levels of creation. Within these exist many subtle levels, but we are unaware of them because our sensory apparatus is not refined enough to locate them.

Yoga teaches that not only do these subtle levels of creation exist but that subtler than the subtlest lies the Self. The only way to experience this absolute consciousness is to refine the mind's ability to perceive.

In meditation a suitable sense object is selected as the focus of attention *(pratyaya)*. As each subtler level of the object is appreciated, so mental activity also becomes more refined, more subtle. The two go together. In this way the attention is led progressively through the levels of thinking, feeling, intellect, and ego, as the object of meditation is appreciated in its finer values.

Eventually the finest level of the object is experienced and, correspondingly, the most refined level of mental activity is attained. When even this movement is transcended, mental activity comes to a complete standstill. The mind thus ceases to exist as an individual entity and merges back into its source, universal consciousness, as a wave falls back into the sea. This consciousness is absolute. Therefore it is beyond both the subjective and objective states of existence, because these are, by definition, relative. For the Self to shine forth, both the subjective—the activity of the mind—and the objective—the mind's object—have to be transcended. This is done by allowing the process of meditation to refine them out of existence.

This is what Patanjali means when he says: "Experience of the finer levels of the senses establishes the settled mind" (1.35). We can transcend mental activity by using any of the senses. The Tibetan Buddhists, for example, have developed many techniques of visualization in order to transcend through the sense of sight. One technique is to focus attention for some time on an object, usually a *mandala* or painting of a deity, and then the eyes are closed and the inner image is experienced in an increasingly refined manner, until it is eventually transcended. Icons are used in a similar way in Christian Orthodox churches. Whichever sense we use, however, the process is the same. Awareness must reach the limit of that particular sense, and then go beyond.

The easiest sense to refine is the sense of hearing. Hearing is the senior sense; it operates through the medium of space *(ākāsha),* which, as we have seen, is the subtlest of the great elements *(panchamahābhūta)* and the one from which the other four—air, fire, water, earth—sequentially unfold, and in which they inhere. It is the first sense to awaken in the fetus, and the last to leave at the time of death—hence the universal tradition of reading sacred scriptures to the dying or recently "dead." Thus the most effective medium for leading the mind to its source is sound, and thinking is a subtly internalized form of sound. The thought, or sound, that is used in meditation is the *mantra*—literally "mind-instrument." This *mantra* is not considered important for its meaning, because preoccupation with this would hold the attention on the level of thinking or feeling, at the surface of the mind. The *mantra* is a vehicle that allows the mind to settle down to a more refined level of activity. The *mantra,* and the procedure for using it correctly, must be learned from a properly qualified teacher.

The process of transcending is a perfectly natural one. It is the result of the mind's desire for greater fulfillment. The Victorian poet Tennyson wrote in the nineteenth century of an experience of transcending he had had quite innocently at different times in his life. "This has come upon me through repeating my own name to myself silently till all at once, as it were out of the intensity of the consciousness of individuality, individuality itself seemed to dissolve and fade away into boundless being, and this not a confused state but the clearest, the surest of the surest, utterly beyond words—where death was an almost laughable impossibility—the loss of personality (if so it were) seeming no extinction but the only true life."

The progressive stages of this settling of the mind are described in *sūtras* 17 and 18 of the first chapter. *Sūtra* 17 describes the four general stages of *samprajñāta samādhi* "settledness with activity" as gross activity, subtle activity, the thrill of bliss as the individual mind expands, and then the state of pure "I-AM-ness." This last state is described at its most refined level in *sūtra* 18:

> After the repeated experience of the settling and ceasing of mental activity comes another *samādhi*. In this only the latent impressions of past experience remain.

The nineteenth verse of Chapter 6 of the *Bhagavad Gītā* refers to the mind as it is described in *sūtra* 18 as being "like a lamp that does not flicker in a wind-less place." A living enlightened master has commented on this:

> As long as the mind is associated with the object, so long it is the experiencing mind; but when the object of experience has diminished to the point where it has disappeared, the mind ceases to be the experiencing mind. Conscious mind becomes consciousness. But during this process of transformation, it first gains the state of its own pure individuality. It is interesting to see that . . . the Sanskrit word used is *chitta,* which signifies that aspect of mind which is a quiet and silent collection of impressions, or seeds of desires. *Chitta* is like water without ripples. It is called *manas,* mind, when ripples arise. When the mind gains this state of *chitta* . . . then it stands steady, like "a lamp which does not flicker in a windless place." It holds its individuality in the void—the abstract fullness around it—because there is nothing for it to experience. It remains undisturbed, awake in itself.
>
> —MAHARISHI MAHESH YOGI

The *Gītā* calls this the state of "resolute intellect." It is the subtlest level of individuality, what Tennyson intuited as "the intensity of the consciousness of individuality." The trinity of experiencer, experiencing,

and object of experience has been left behind, and
the pure intellect is like a silent wave, poised to fall
back into the silent sea of the Self.

The Siddhis

The third chapter of the *Yoga Sūtras* deals with what
may seem to be the most fantastic aspect of Patanjali's
teaching: the *siddhis.* The word *siddhi* means "perfec-
tion, accomplishment, complete success"—nouns that
derive from its original meaning as an archery term
signifying "hitting the target dead center." (Interest-
ingly, the Greek word *harmartia,* translated as "sin" in
the New Testament, was also originally a term used
in archery, meaning "missing the mark.") *Siddhi* is used
to describe the so-called supernormal powers that
come to the expanded mind. Patanjali is not the only
authority to mention these powers; the *Linga Purāna,*
Agni Purāna, and *Shiva Sūtras* all spend considerable
time discussing them, as do many Buddhist texts, particularly those of the Tibetan schools. At a more popular level, the epic legends of the *Rāmāyana* and the
Mahābhārata describe the great heroes of antiquity
employing the *siddhis* in their cosmic escapades.

Nor are these *siddhis* confined to the mysterious
East. The Western religious traditions also contain
many accounts of them—Noah, Elijah, Isaiah, and,

of course, Jesus himself were all accredited with miraculous abilities. So were the philosophers Socrates and Apollonius. In more recent history such saints as Catherine of Siena, Teresa of Avila, and Joseph of Copertino all displayed supernormal powers, and in the unlikely setting of Victorian England the young Scot D. D. Home caused a sensation by correctly foretelling future events, making musical instruments play with nobody near them, increasing or diminishing his height by eight inches, and levitating both himself and others many feet into the air.

How are we to understand and evaluate such extraordinary phenomena that, according to the *Yoga Sūtras,* include the ability to become invisible, materialize objects, and understand the sounds of all living beings?

The *siddhis* are the result of practicing what Patanjali calls *sanyama* (coherence). He defines this as "*dhāranā, dhyāna,* and *samādhi* practiced together" (3.4). We have seen that the techniques of yoga settle the body and the breathing, and this allows the senses to retire as the mind settles down in meditation. Mental activity becomes more and more refined until it eventually disappears altogether in transcendental consciousness. The key word here is "eventually." This settling proceeds by stages; it is a gradual progression from normal thinking to a state of total silence. *Sanyama* is the technique of allowing a thought to be entertained by the mind at the very threshold of unbounded consciousness. At this profound level the mind, "its essential nature shining forth in purity, is as if unbounded" (3.3). The qualification "as if" is important here, because "even *sanyama* is outside that pure unboundedness" (3.8). This is the subtlest level of the individual thinking mind.

This delicate threshold area was defined in the first chapter as *ritambharā,* "where consciousness perceives only the truth" (1.48). Here the mind is at its most powerful. Mind is like light; the nearer its source, the stronger it is. *Ritambharā* is that level where the individual mind still exists in a concentrated form. All the power of consciousness, that reservoir of intelligence that is the source of all thought, is at its disposal. The mind is like a drawn bow; there is tremendous potential energy. Releasing the arrow of thought so that it swiftly and unerringly "hits the target dead center" is *siddhi.*

When the mind is this refined, it imbibes many of the qualities of its source, like a wave with all the weight of the ocean behind it. Consciousness is omnipresent and eternal, Patanjali tells us. In *sanyama* the mind is almost as unrestricted, and thought is no longer limited by those boundaries, which, in everyday experience, seem insurmountable. Thus a mind directed in *sanyama* can know the past and future because it is drawing on an area of life that is beyond time; it can "see what is subtle, hidden from view or far away" because it operates from a level that is beyond the limitations of space; it can see the future consequences of past action because it has transcended causality. If a mind is pure enough to operate consciously from this level, there is nothing it cannot accomplish.

Such far-reaching conclusions, which seem to contradict all known physical laws, may appear to belong to the realms of infantile fantasy. Yet it is important to remember that science (unlike religious belief, incidentally) is embedded in uncertainty, and the currently accepted laws of science are not in themselves absolute. Not only may they be transcended as greater understanding of the nature of reality dawns—Einstein's relativity theory was superseded a mere couple of years after it was articulated by the advent of quantum theory—but even in their own time they do not claim to be more than a workable approximation of the truth. Strictly speaking, any physical law is statistical, an approximate law—rule even—that has its basis in the probable occurrence of a series of microscopic events. Furthermore, the activities of the gross, or surface, levels of life, explicable by the classical laws of physics, are themselves dependent on, and may even be contradicted by, the laws operating at a subtler level. Thus, matter, relatively stable and solid at its surface, is revealed to be a vortex of whirling energy at the atomic level, and at an even deeper level this energy gives way to open space and mere potential. Indeed, the latest research into the subtlest levels of matter, the subatomic universe that is the province of quantum physics, reveals a reality that is every bit as strange as Patanjali's.

Quantum theory is a central pillar of modern physics. It has been responsible for our understanding of chemical bonding, the structure of atoms, molecules, and nuclear reactions, and has led to many of the most recent developments in technology: lasers, electron microscopes, and nuclear power. It has also dealt the death-blow to many of our commonsense notions about matter, space, time, and reality.

Niels Bohr, one of the originators of the theory, declared that it is meaningless to regard any atom or subatomic particle as really existing in a particular condition before we observe it. Only within the context of an actual experiment does a reality appear. If the experiment is changed, so is the reality. Indeed, it is not even possible to regard atoms as *things,* i.e., existing in a well-defined state, independent of our perception of them. In other words, at this level the consciousness of the observer is crucial in influencing, even creating, what is observed.

What is more, quantum field theory tells us that at the heart of creation lies "the vacuum state." This is a state of perfect order, or zero entropy. It is beyond all boundaries of time and space, and, as the empty source of all light and matter in the universe, an area of pure potential. All particles of matter are "excitations" of this abstract ground state. It is the state of least excitation, which is nevertheless equally present in all excited states. The vacuum state is thus an exact objective counterpart to the yogi's subjective experience of the Self.

The closer we get to this vacuum state, the less the old laws of classical physics apply. At this level, life is a field of "all possibilities." Anything can happen. Subatomic particles appear out of nowhere and then disappear again; they tunnel through impenetrable barriers or inexplicably reverse direction. The vacuum state can quite possibly be the source of an infinite number of separate realities, parallel universes, each with its own characteristics.

A simple example of this is the behavior of liquid

helium. Thermodynamics tells us that as temperature decreases in a system, so does disorder. When the temperature of liquid helium is lowered to just above "absolute zero" (−275° C), it enters an utterly flat, silent, and stable state, and becomes "superfluid." As there is no disorder among the constituent atoms of superfluid helium, it can enjoy what is known as "frictionless flow."

This ability to flow has some startling manifestations. If a glassful of ordinary liquid is removed from a container and held above it, the liquid cannot by itself return to the container. But if the same is done with superfluid helium, it cannot be contained. Because of its supernormal power of flow, it will spontaneously climb out of the glass, in a layer one atom thick, and rejoin the rest of the helium in the container below. From the standpoint of classical physics, this is impossible. It cannot logically happen because it contravenes the established laws. Yet it does!

We can see the analogy between the phenomenon of superfluidity and what Patanjali says is possible for the least excited state of awareness, the Self. The yogi is able to operate from the silent and stable area of the mind that is almost universal. The *siddhis* are the art of letting this level of mind consciously flow into thought, the science of introducing a conscious intention at the most delicate, coherent, and unified level of awareness. This intention, operating at the microscopic level, can overturn the laws operating at a grosser level, thus creating what we conventionally call miracles. But all of this, it must be repeated, is quite "natural"; a *siddhi* is just the utilization of natural principles and laws to translate the energy of one level of reality, more essential and powerful, to another. Through this technique, the yogi can influence his own body and his environment—either immediate or at a distance—and his sense perception can be expanded far beyond its normal range, for the Self is as much "there" as "here"—it is omnipresent. Having the knowledge of the cosmos within his own Being, he enjoys subjectively what we are beginning to realize is objectively possible.

Only a mind that has been purified by the eight limbs of yoga will be able to perform *sanyama* with any effect. The *siddhis* cannot be performed with any negative or selfish intent, because such feelings cannot be maintained at this fine level. Moreover, Patanjali agrees with the other great teachers when he emphasizes that the *siddhis* are not to be practiced for their own sake, or as a means to increase personal power; they are not weapons in the armory of egocentric magic. Ultimately, the *siddhis* are useful only because they nurture Enlightenment, and "*sanyama* has its application at every stage of the development of this supreme knowledge" (3.6). We are specifically told that *siddhis* "are subordinate to the pure unboundedness but are the perfections of a mind still operating at the subtle level" (3.37).

The teaching on the transformations *(parināma* 3.9–11) explains how the *siddhis* lead to freedom. By *sanyama* the value of fully expanded awareness is, as it were, coaxed into the very fabric of the thinking mind, so that proficiency in the technique leaves the mind saturated with silence, no matter how active it may be on the surface. *Sanyama* results in "the state in which activity and silence are equally balanced in the mind" (3.12). When this balance is permanent, there is Enlightenment.

It should be clearly understood that the present translation is in no way intended as an instruction in the *siddhis*. The technique of *sanyama,* like meditation itself, is a delicate one, and can only be learned personally from a qualified teacher. It can never be learned from books. Moreover, the actual translation of any particular *sūtra* in the present version is only one way among many that the *sūtra* could be rendered. The *Yoga Sūtras,* like all scriptures, operate on different levels of meaning at the same time, by exploiting the ambiguities inherent in language. Sanskrit is particularly well-suited to this device, which it calls "the twilight language" *(sandhyā bhāshā)*. The extent to which the full subtlety of a particular *sūtra* is revealed depends on the consciousness of the interpreter, which is why no translation can ever be a substitute for the living teaching expounded by an enlightened being.

In this translation I have consulted what seems to me to be the two most acute commentaries: those of Vyāsa and Vijnāna Bhikshu. Even these disagree in their interpretation of many of the *sūtras*. Working in such exalted company, I am only too well aware that the depth of my subject outstrips my ability to fathom it!

One last word: Do, wherever possible, read the *Yoga Sūtras* aloud. The teaching of yoga is an aural tradition, which knows the ability of sound to transform the hearer. We live in a cacophonous age and have forgotten the power of the right sound to heal and regenerate. But the *sūtras* date from an age of preliterate innocence, when each word uttered by the bard or seer possessed a tremendous and mysterious creative power—the ability to penetrate deeply into consciousness and plant the seeds of fresh perception. It was a time when "the Word was with God and the Word was God," so much so that even the timely hearing of certain scriptures was said to confer liberation.

The *sūtras* were passed down by word of mouth for centuries before they were committed to writing. Like the *Vedas* and *Upanishads* before them, they have been chanted, sung, and murmured for thousands of years, reverberating around cave sanctuaries, temple halls, and centers of learning and pilgrimage. Every sound has its effect, and a pure sound will carry the mind to that silence which is the source of all sounds. This ability to transport the listener is not wholly confined to the original Sanskrit; even in translation, some of the resonance can be transmitted. For all their restrained logic and classical purity, the *Yoga Sūtras* are a hymn of praise, which should be recited far and wide for all to hear. We are in dire need of their wisdom, for it is in the understanding and utilization of the precious gift of human conscious-ness that our next evolutionary advance lies.

Laxfield, Suffolk, England
2001

THE YOGA SUTRAS

OF PATANJALI

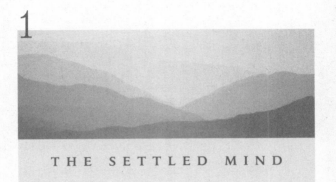

1

THE SETTLED MIND

1.　And now the teaching on yoga begins.

2.　Yoga is the settling of the mind into silence.

3.　When the mind has settled, we are
　　established in our essential nature, which
　　is unbounded consciousness.

4.　Our essential nature is usually overshadowed
　　by the activity of the mind.

5.　There are five types of mental activity.
　　They may or may not cause suffering.

6.　These five are:
　　　understanding,
　　　misunderstanding,
　　　imagination,

sleep,
and memory.

7. Understanding is correct knowledge based
on direct perception, inference, or the
reliable testimony of others.

8. Misunderstanding is the delusion that stems
from a false impression of reality.

9. Imagination is thought based on an image
conjured up by words, and is without
substance.

10. Sleep is the mental activity that has as its
content the sense of nothingness.

11. And memory is the returning to the mind of
past experience.

12. These five types of mental activity are settled
through the practice of yoga and the
freedom it bestows.

THE SETTLED MIND

13. The practice of yoga is the commitment to become established in the state of freedom.

14. The practice of yoga will be firmly rooted when it is maintained consistently and with dedication over a long period.

15. Freedom is that triumphant state of consciousness that is beyond the influence of desire.
   The mind ceases to thirst for anything it has seen or heard of; even what is promised in the scriptures.

16. And supreme freedom is that complete liberation from the world of change that comes of knowing the unbounded Self.

17. The settled mind is known as *samādhi*.
   In *samprajnāta samādhi,* the settled state is accompanied by mental activity:

           first on the gross level,
           then on the subtle level,
           then a feeling of bliss,
           and finally the sense of pure "I-AM-ness."

18. After the repeated experience of the settling and ceasing of mental activity comes another *samādhi*.
In this only the latent impressions of past experience remain.

19. This is the nature of existence for beings without gross physical bodies and for those who are absorbed in the womb of all life awaiting rebirth.

20. For others this *samādhi* is preceded by trust, perseverance, recollection, tranquillity, and wisdom.

21. It is near for those who ardently desire it.

22. Yet even among them there are degrees— mild, moderate, and intense.

23. It can also come from complete surrender to the almighty Lord.

⊞

24. The Lord is a unique being who exists beyond all suffering.
Unblemished by action, He is free from both its cause and its effects.

25. In Him lies the finest seed of all knowledge.

26. Being beyond time, He is the Teacher of even the most ancient tradition of teachers.

27. He is expressed through the sound of the sacred syllable *OM*.

28. It should be repeated and its essence realized.

29. Then the mind will turn inward and the obstacles that stand in the way of progress will disappear.

⊞

30. These obstacles are:
        illness,
        fatigue,
        doubt,
        carelessness,
        laziness,
        attachment,
        delusion,
        the failure to achieve *samādhi,*
        and the failure to maintain *samādhi.*
     They are distractions from the path of yoga.

31. Such distractions make the body restless, the
     breathing coarse, and the mind agitated.
     They result in suffering.

32. But they can be eliminated if the mind is
     repeatedly brought to a single focus.

33. The mind becomes clear and serene when
     the qualities of the heart are cultivated:

       friendliness toward the joyful,
       compassion toward the suffering,
       happiness toward the pure,
       and impartiality toward the impure.

34. Or through the practice of various breathing exercises.

35. Experience of the finer levels of the senses establishes the settled mind.

36. So does experience of the inner radiance that is free from sorrow.

37. So does being attuned to another mind that is itself unperturbed by desire.

38. So does witnessing the process of dreaming or dreamless sleep.

39. So does any meditation that is held in high esteem.

40. The sovereignty of the mind that is settled,
    extends from the smallest of the small to the
    greatest of the great.

41. As a flawless crystal absorbs what is placed
    before it, so the settled mind is transparent
    to whatever it meets—the seer, the process
    of seeing, or the object seen.
    This is *samāpatti*—the state of mental
    absorption.

42. The first stage of absorption is when the object
    of attention is gross, and its name and other
    thoughts are mingled together in the mind.

43. The second stage is when the memory is
    purified and the mind is quiet enough to be
    absorbed in the object of attention.

44. In the same way the third and fourth stages
    of absorption are explained: these occur
    when the object of attention is subtle.

⊞

45. The range of subtle objects includes all the levels of creation, extending to the limit of the *gunas*.

46. These levels of *samādhi* are concerned only with external objects.

47. But on refinement of the fourth stage of absorption, there is the dawning of the spiritual light of the Self.

48. This level is *ritambharā,* where consciousness perceives only the truth.

⊞

49. The knowledge gained through *ritambharā* is qualitatively different from that gained in the usual way through testimony and inference. The former means is intuitive and sees things as they are in their totality, whereas the latter means is partial.

50. The impression born of *ritambharā* prevents
    the accumulation of further latent impressions.

51. And when even the latent impression of
    ritambharā has been brought to a settled
    state, then all activity ceases and *nirbīja
    samādhi*—the unbounded consciousness of
    the Self—alone remains.

2

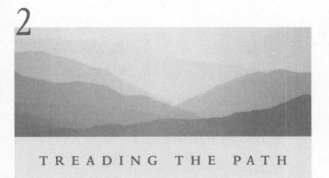

TREADING THE PATH

1. Purification,
    refinement,
    surrender.
    These are the practical steps on the path of
    yoga.

2. They nourish the state of *samādhi* and weaken
    the causes of suffering.

3. The causes of suffering are five:
    ignorance of our real nature,
    egoism,
    attachment,
    aversion,
    and the fear of death, which makes us
    cling to life.

4. Ignorance of our real nature is the source of the other four, whether they be dormant, weak, suspended, or fully active.

5. Ignorance is the failure to discriminate between the permanent and the impermanent, the pure and the impure, bliss and suffering, the Self and the non-Self.

6. Egoism, the limiting sense of "I," results from the individual intellect's attributing the power of consciousness to itself.

7. Attachment is clinging to pleasure.

8. Aversion is clinging to pain.

9. And the fear of death is a spontaneous feeling, deeply rooted in us all, no matter how learned we may be.

10. The subtle causes of suffering are destroyed
when the mind merges back into the
unmanifest.

11. The gross effects of suffering are discarded
through meditation.

12. The impressions of past action, stored deep
in the mind, are the seeds of desire.
They ripen into action in seen and unseen
ways—if not in this life, then in a future one.

13. As long as action leaves its seed in the mind,
this seed will grow, generating more births,
more lives, more actions.

14. In these too, the fruit of wrong action is
sorrow, the fruit of right action is joy.

15. Life is uncertain, change causes fear, and
latent impressions bring pain—all is indeed
suffering to one who has developed
discrimination.

16. But the suffering yet to come should be
averted.

17. The cause of suffering is that the unbounded
Self is overshadowed by the world.

18. The world is the play of the *gunas*—
the universal energies of light, motion,
and mass.
They take form as the elements and the
senses.
The purpose of the world is to provide us
with experience and thus to lead us to
liberation.

19. The *gunas* operate on various levels:
    gross,
    subtle,
    causal,
    and unmanifest.

20. But the Self is boundless.
    It is the pure consciousness that illumines the contents of the mind.

21. It is only for the sake of the Self that the world exists.

❖

22. Although the limitations of the world disappear for one who knows the Self, they are not destroyed, because they continue to exist for others.

23. The Self is obscured by the world in order that the reality of both may be discovered.

24. It is ignorance of our real nature that causes the Self to be obscured.

25. When ignorance is destroyed, the Self is liberated from its identification with the world.
    This liberation is Enlightenment.

❖

26. Ignorance is destroyed by the undisturbed discrimination between the Self and the world.

27. There are seven stages in the growth of this wisdom.

28. The distinction between pure consciousness and the world is revealed by the light of knowledge, when the nervous system has been purified by the practice of yoga.

29. There are eight limbs of yoga:
    yama—the laws of life,
    niyama—the rules for living,
    āsana—the physical postures,
    prānāyāma—the breathing exercises,
    pratyāhāra—the retirement of the senses,
    dhāranā—steadiness of mind,
    dhyāna—meditation,
    samādhi—the settled mind.

30. The laws of life are five:
    nonviolence,

truthfulness,
integrity,
chastity,
nonattachment.

31. These laws are universal.
    Unaffected by time, place, birth, or
    circumstance, together they constitute
    the "Great Law of Life."

32. The rules for living are five:
    simplicity,
    contentment,
    purification,
    refinement,
    surrender to the Lord.

33. When negative feelings restrict us, the
    opposite should be cultivated.

34. Negative feelings, such as violence, are
    damaging to life, whether we act upon

them ourselves, or cause or condone them
in others.
They are born of greed, anger, or delusion,
and may be slight, moderate, or intense.
Their fruit is endless ignorance and suffering.
To remember this is to cultivate the opposite.

35. When we are firmly established in
    nonviolence, all beings around us cease
    to feel hostility.

36. When we are firmly established in truthfulness,
    action accomplishes its desired end.

37. When we are firmly established in integrity,
    all riches present themselves freely.

38. When we are firmly established in chastity,
    subtle potency is generated.

39. When we are established in nonattachment,
    the nature and purpose of existence is
    understood.

40. Simplicity destroys identification with the body, and brings freedom from contact with other bodies.

41. Purity of mind, cheerfulness, mastery of the senses, one-pointedness, and readiness for Self-realization follow.

42. From contentment, unsurpassed happiness is gained.

43. By purification, the body and the senses are perfected.

44. Refinement brings communion with the desired celestial being.

45. From surrender to the Lord, the state of *samādhi* is perfected.

46. The physical postures should be steady and comfortable.

47. They are mastered when all effort is relaxed
and the mind is absorbed in the Infinite.

48. Then we are no longer upset by the play of
opposites.

❖

49. Next come the breathing exercises, which
suspend the flow of breath and increase the
life energy.

50. The life energy is increased by regulation of
the out-breath, the in-breath, or the breath
in mid-flow.
Depending upon the volume, and the length
and frequency of holding, the breathing
becomes slow and refined.

51. The fourth kind of *prānāyāma* takes us
beyond the domain of inner and outer.

❖

52. Then the light of the intellect is unveiled.

53. And the mind is prepared for steadiness.

54. The senses retire from their objects by following the natural inward movement of the mind.

55. From this comes supreme mastery of the senses.

3

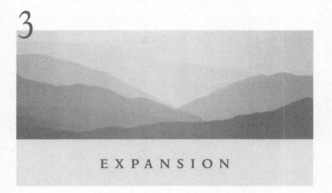

EXPANSION

1. When the attention is held focused on an object, this is known as *dhāranā*.

2. When awareness flows evenly toward the point of attention, this is known as *dhyāna*.

3. And when that same awareness, its essential nature shining forth in purity, is as if unbounded, this is known as *samādhi*.

4. *Dhāranā, dhyāna,* and *samādhi* practiced together are known as *sanyama*.

5. When *sanyama* is mastered, the light of supreme knowledge dawns.

6. But *sanyama* has its application at every stage of the development of this knowledge.

7. It is the heart of yoga, more intimate than the preceding limits.

8. Yet even *sanyama* is outside that pure unboundedness.

9. *Nirodha parināma,* the transformation of the bounded state, occurs when the attention moves from the rise and fall of the mind's impressions to the silence that pervades when its activity is settled.

10. This silence flows evenly into the mind, because it becomes a latent impression itself.

11. *Samādhi parināma,* the transformation of the settled state, is the alternation between the mind's being one-pointed and its being unbounded.

12. And from this comes *ekāgratā parināma,* the transformation of one-pointedness, the state

in which activity and silence are equally
balanced in the mind.

⊞

13. These are the transformations of the mind.
The transformations that operate in matter—
transformations of quality, form, and state—
are similarly explained.

14. Each object carries its past, present, and
future qualities within it.

15. The diversity of matter is caused by the laws
of nature which conduct evolution.

16. *Sanyama* on the three transformations brings
knowledge of the past and future.

⊞

17. Perception of an object is usually confused,
because its name, its form, and an idea about
it are all superimposed upon each other.
By doing *sanyama* on the distinction between

these three, we can understand the sound of all living beings.

18. From the direct experience of latent impressions comes knowledge of previous births.

19. And from the direct experience of its state, we can know the quality of another mind.

20. We know the quality, but not the content of the mind, because that is not within the sphere of this *sanyama*.

⊞

21. *Sanyama* on the form of the body makes it imperceptible, by breaking the contact between the eye of the observer and the light reflected by the body.
From this *sanyama* invisibility comes.

22. The fruits of an action may return to the doer quickly or slowly.
From *sanyama* on the fruit of an action comes

foreknowledge of the time of death, and the understanding of omens.

23. From *sanyama* on friendliness, compassion, and happiness, these qualities blossom.

24. From *sanyama* on the strength of an elephant, or other creatures, we gain that strength.

25. By directing the inner light we can see what is subtle, hidden from view or far away.

26. From *sanyama* on the sun comes knowledge of the various realms of the universe.

27. From *sanyama* on the moon comes knowledge of the arrangement of the stars.

28. From *sanyama* on the pole star comes knowledge of their motion.

29. *Sanyama* on the navel center brings knowledge of the bodily system.

30. *Sanyama* on the hollow in the throat brings cessation of hunger and thirst.

31. *Sanyama* on the *kūrma* nerve in the trachea brings steadiness.

32. From *sanyama* on the light in the head, we see the perfected ones.

33. By the clarity of intuitive perception everything can be known.

34. From *sanyama* on the heart comes awareness of pure mind.

⊞

35. The Self and the contents of the mind are completely separate.
    Our usual experience, which is directed to outer fulfillment, fails to distinguish between them.

Sanyama on inner fulfillment brings knowledge of the Self.

36. From this are born intuitive clarity, and finest hearing, finest touch, finest sight, finest taste, and finest smell.

37. These are subordinate to the state of pure unboundedness, but are the perfections of a mind still operating at the subtle level.

38. When attachment to the body is loosened and there is perfect knowledge of the movement of the mind, the ability to enter another's body is gained.

39. On mastery of *udāna,* the life breath that rises through the body, we can direct it upward and avoid contact with such things as water, mud, and thorns.

40. On mastery of *samāna,* the life breath that nourishes the body, the body shines with radiant light.

41. From *sanyama* on the relationship of hearing and *ākāsha,* celestial hearing is gained.

42. From *sanyama* on the relationship between body and *ākāsha,* together with absorption in the lightness of cotton fiber, we can move through the air at will.

43. The operation of the mind outside the confines of the body is known as *mahāvidehā*—"the great state beyond the body."
    This destroys the veil that covers the light of discrimination.

44. Mastery over the elements comes from *sanyama* on their forms—
    earth, water, fire, air, and space;
    on their characteristics—
    mass, fluidity, heat, motion, and omnipresence;

on their essences—

odor, flavor, form, texture, and sound;
on the relationship between these forms,
characteristics, and essences and on their
evolutionary purpose.

45. From mastery over the elements come the
eight physical perfections:
shrinking the body to the size of an atom,
becoming very light,
becoming very heavy,
becoming very large,
developing an irresistible will,
controlling the elements,
materializing objects and causing them
to disappear,
fulfilling all desires.
In addition, the body becomes perfected and
cannot be harmed by its own mortality.

46. The attributes of a perfected body are beauty,
grace, strength, and adamantine hardness.

47. Mastery over the senses is gained from
    sanyama
    on their power of perceiving;
    on the sense organs themselves;
    on the feeling of "I-ness" which sense
        perception creates;
    on the relationship between these aspects
        of the senses
    and on their evolutionary purpose.

48. As a result of this, the senses can move with
    the speed of thought and operate
    independently of the body.
    This is mastery over Nature.

49. He who has realized the distinction between
    the subtlest level of his mind, which is
    translucent intellect, and the Self, enjoys
    supremacy over all creation.
    Nothing remains unknown to him.

50. And when he is unattached even to this state, the very seeds of bondage are destroyed, and Enlightenment follows.

51. We should not respond with pleasure or pride to the alluring invitations of celestial beings, because this will obstruct progress, and it is always possible to fall.

52. From *sanyama* on moments and their succession, the finest discriminative knowledge is born.

53. This enables us to distinguish between two objects that are to all appearances identical.

54. Knowledge born of the finest discrimination takes us to the farthest shore.
    It is intuitive, omniscient, and beyond all divisions of time and space.

55. And when the translucent intellect is as pure as the Self, there is Self Realization.

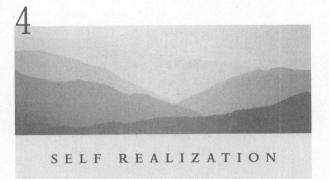

4

SELF REALIZATION

1. The perfections may already be present at birth, or they can be developed by herbs, *mantras,* by purification, and by *samādhi.*

2. Any change into a new state of being is the result of the fullness of Nature unfolding inherent potential.

3. But the apparent causes of a change do not in fact bring it about.
   They merely remove the obstacles to natural growth, as a farmer clears the ground for his crops.

4. All minds are created by ego—the separative sense of "I."

5. All these expressions of individuality, however highly developed, are the impulses of the force of evolution.

6. And of these, only the mind born of meditation is free from the latent impressions that generate desire.

7. The actions of an enlightened being are neither black nor white, but those of others are threefold.

8. From their actions are sown the seeds of mental tendencies that bear fruit appropriate to their nature.

9. Memory and impression have similar forms. They give birth to our tendencies, which operate continuously to shape our lives, even if their cause is separated from their effect by time, by place, or by lifetimes.

10. And tendencies are without beginning, because the desire for fulfillment, which sustains them, is everlasting.

11. They are maintained by the mind's bondage to its objects, through the cycle of cause and effect.

⊞

12. The past and the future exist within an object, and are due to the difference in the characteristics of that object.

13. Manifested characteristics are the present; unmanifested, the past and future.
    All are the workings of the *gunas*.

14. The state of an object at any moment arises from the unique state of the *gunas* then operating.

15. Two similar objects appear different because of the difference in the minds that perceive them.

16. An object does not depend on a single mind for its existence, for if it did, what

would become of it when not perceived by
that mind?

※

17. An object is experienced only when it colors
the mind.

18. But the mind itself is always experienced
because it is witnessed by the unchanging
Self.

19. The mind does not shine by its own light.
It too is an object, illumined by the Self.

20. Not being self-luminous, the mind cannot
be aware of its object and itself at the
same time.

21. Nor is the mind illumined by another more
subtle mind, for that would imply the
absurdity of an infinite series of minds, and
the resulting confusion of memories.

※

22. When the unmoving consciousness of the
Self assumes the form of intellect, it becomes
conscious mind.

23. The mind that is colored by both its object
and the Self, is all-embracing.

24. And the mind, despite its countless separative
tendencies, exists for the sake of the Self,
because it is dependent upon it.

25. All confusion about the nature of the Self
vanishes for one who has seen its glory.

26. Then, truly, the mind begins to experience
the Self as separate from activity, and is
naturally drawn toward Enlightenment.

27. All thoughts that arise to interrupt this
discrimination are born of the latent
impressions that still exist.

28. These are to be destroyed by the same means as were described for the causes of suffering.

29. One who has attained complete discrimination between the subtlest level of mind and the Self has no higher knowledge to acquire. This is *dharma megha samādhi*—the state of Unclouded Truth.

30. It destroys the causes of suffering, and the bondage of action disappears.

31. Knowledge that has been freed from the veils of impurity is unbounded. Whatever can be known is insignificant in its light.

32. This *samādhi* completes the transformations of the *gunas* and fulfills the purpose of evolution.

33. Now the process by which evolution unfolds through time is understood.

34. The *gunas,* their purpose fulfilled, return to their original state of harmony, and pure unbounded consciousness remains, forever established in its own absolute nature. This is Enlightenment.

ALISTAIR SHEARER did postgraduate work in Sanskrit at the University of Lancaster after studying literature at Cambridge. He has practiced and taught meditation for many years. He currently divides his time between lecturing and writing on the sacred art of Hinduism and Buddhism, teaching meditation courses, and leading cultural tours to the Indian subcontinent each winter (www.trishulatravel.com). His latest publications include *The Spirit of Asia* and *Buddha: The Intelligent Heart*.

OTHER BELL TOWER BOOKS

*Books that nourish the soul, illuminate the mind,
and speak directly to the heart*

Rob Baker
PLANNING MEMORIAL CELEBRATIONS
A Sourcebook

A one-stop handbook for a situation more and more of us are
facing as we grow older. / 0-609-80404-9 · *Softcover*

Thomas Berry
THE GREAT WORK
Our Way into the Future

The grandfather of Deep Ecology teaches us how to move
from a human-centered view of the world to one focused on
the earth and all its inhabitants.
0-609-80499-5 · *Softcover*

Cynthia Bourgeault
LOVE IS STRONGER THAN DEATH
The Mystical Union of Two Souls

Both the story of the incandescent love between two hermits
and a guidebook for those called to this path of soulwork.
0-609-60473-2 · *Hardcover*

Madeline Bruser
THE ART OF PRACTICING
Making Music from the Heart

A classic work on how to practice music that combines meditative principles with information on body mechanics and medicine.

0-609-80177-5 · *Softcover*

Thomas Byrom (Trans.)
THE DHAMMAPADA
The Sayings of the Buddha

The first book in a series of small spiritual classics entitled Sacred Teachings.

0-609-60888-6 · *Hardcover*

Melody Ermachild Chavis
ALTARS IN THE STREET
A Courageous Memoir of Community and Spiritual Awakening

A deeply moving account that captures the essence of human struggles and resourcefulness.

0-609-80196-1 · *Softcover*

Marc David
NOURISHING WISDOM
A Mind/Body Approach to Nutrition and Well-Being

A book that advocates awareness in eating.

0-517-88129-2 · *Softcover*

Kat Duff
THE ALCHEMY OF ILLNESS
A luminous inquiry into the function and purpose
of illness.
0-609-89943-0 · *Softcover*

Joan Furman, M.S.N., R.N., and David McNabb
THE DYING TIME
*Practical Wisdom for the Dying
and Their Caregivers*
A comprehensive guide, filled with physical, emotional,
and spiritual advice.
0-609-80003-5 · *Softcover*

Bernard Glassman
BEARING WITNESS
A Zen Master's Lessons in Making Peace
How Glassman started the Zen Peacemaker Order and what
each of us can do to make peace in our hearts and in the world.
0-609-80391-3 · *Softcover*

Bernie Glassman and Rick Fields
INSTRUCTIONS TO THE COOK
*A Zen Master's Lessons in Living a Life
that Matters*
A distillation of Zen wisdom that can be used equally well as a
manual on business or spiritual practice, cooking or life.
0-517-88829-7 · *Softcover*

Niles Elliot Goldstein
GOD AT THE EDGE
*Searching for the Divine in Uncomfortable
and Unexpected Places*

A book about adventure, raw experience, and facing
inner demons.
0-609-80488-X · *Softcover*

Burghild Nina Holzer
A WALK BETWEEN HEAVEN AND EARTH
A Personal Journal on Writing and the Creative Process

How keeping a journal focuses and expands our awareness of
ourselves and everything that touches our lives.
0-517-88096-2 · *Softcover*

Greg Johanson and Ron Kurtz
GRACE UNFOLDING
Psychotherapy in the Spirit of the Tao-te ching

The interaction of client and therapist illuminated through the
gentle power and wisdom of Lao Tsu's ancient classic.
0-517-88130-6 · *Softcover*

Selected by Marcia and Jack Kelly
ONE HUNDRED GRACES
Mealtime Blessings

A collection of graces from many traditions, inscribed in callig-
raphy reminiscent of the manuscripts of medieval Europe.
0-609-80093-0 · *Softcover*

Jack and Marcia Kelly
SANCTUARIES
*A Guide to Lodgings in Monasteries, Abbeys,
and Retreats of the United States*

For those in search of renewal and a little peace;
described by the *New York Times* as "the *Michelin Guide*
of the retreat set."
0-517-88517-4 · *Softcover*

Lorraine Kisly, ed.
ORDINARY GRACES
Christian Teachings on the Interior Life

An essential collection of the deepest spiritual, religious, and
psychological teachings of Christianity.
0-609-80618-1 · *Softcover*

Barbara Lachman
THE JOURNAL OF HILDEGARD OF BINGEN

A year in the life of the twelfth-century German saint—
the diary she never had the time to write herself.
0-517-88390-2 · *Softcover*

Stephen Levine
A YEAR TO LIVE
How to Live This Year As If It Were Your Last

Using the consciousness of our mortality to enter into
a new and vibrant relationship with life.
0-609-80194-5 · *Softcover*

Helen M. Luke

OLD AGE

Journey into Simplicity

A classic text on how to age wisely by one of the
great Jungian analysts of our time.

0-609-80590-8 · *Softcover*

Helen M. Luke

SUCH STUFF AS DREAMS ARE MADE ON

The Autobiography and Journals of Helen M. Luke

A memoir, 140 pages culled from the 54 volumes of her journals, and 45 black-and-white photos—the summation
of her life and work.

0-609-80589-4 · *Softcover*

Marcia Prager

THE PATH OF BLESSING

Experiencing the Energy and Abundance of the Divine

How to use the traditional Jewish practice of calling down a
blessing on each action as a profound path of spiritual growth.

0-609-80393-X · *Softcover*

Ram Dass and Mirabai Bush

COMPASSION IN ACTION

Setting Out on the Path of Service

Heartfelt encouragement and advice for those ready to commit
time and energy to relieving suffering in the world.

0-517-88520-X · *Softcover*

Saki Santorelli
HEAL THY SELF
Lessons on Mindfulness in Medicine

An invitation to patients and health care professionals
to bring mindfulness into the crucible of the
healing relationship.
0-609-80504-5 · *Softcover*

Rabbi Rami M. Shapiro
MINYAN
Ten Principles for Living a Life of Integrity

A primer for those interested to know what Judaism has
to offer the spiritually hungry.
0-609-80055-8 · *Softcover*

Rabbi Rami M. Shapiro (Trans.)
PROVERBS
The Wisdom of Solomon

The second in a series of small spiritual classics entitled
Sacred Teachings.
0-609-60889-4 · *Hardcover*

Rabbi Rami M. Shapiro
WISDOM OF THE JEWISH SAGES
A Modern Reading of Pirke Avot

A third-century treasury of maxims on justice, integrity, and
virtue—Judaism's principal ethical scripture.
0-517-79966-9 · *Hardcover*

Jean Smith
THE BEGINNER'S GUIDE TO ZEN BUDDHISM

A comprehensive and easily accessible introduction that assumes no prior knowledge of Zen Buddhism.

0-609-80466-9 · *Softcover*

Rabbi Joseph Telushkin
THE BOOK OF JEWISH VALUES
A Day-by-Day Guide to Ethical Living

Ancient and modern advice on how to remain honest in a morally complicated world.

0-609-60330-2 · *Hardcover*

James Thornton
A FIELD GUIDE TO THE SOUL
A Down-to-Earth Handbook of Spiritual Practice

In the tradition of *The Seat of the Soul, The Soul's Code,* and *Care of the Soul,* a primer readers are calling "the Bible for the new millennium."

0-609-80392-1 · *Softcover*

Joan Tollifson
BARE-BONES MEDITATION
Waking Up from the Story of My Life

An unvarnished, exhilarating account of one woman's struggle to make sense of her life.

0-517-88792-4 · *Softcover*

Michael Toms and Justine Willis Toms
TRUE WORK
Doing What You Love and Loving What You Do

Wisdom for the workplace from the husband-and-wife team of
NPR's weekly radio program *New Dimensions*.
0-609-80212-7 · *Softcover*

BUDDHA LAUGHING
A Tricycle Book of Cartoons

A marvelous opportunity for self-reflection for those who tend
to take themselves too seriously. / 0-609-80409-X · *Softcover*

Arinna Weisman and Jean Smith
THE BEGINNER'S GUIDE TO INSIGHT MEDITATION

A primer on Vipassana Buddhism by a prominent teacher and
one of her students. / 0-609-80467-5 · *Softcover*

Richard Whelan, ed.
SELF-RELIANCE
*The Wisdom of Ralph Waldo Emerson as
Inspiration for Daily Living*

A distillation of Emerson's spiritual writings for
contemporary readers. / 0-517-58512-X · *Softcover*

*Bell Tower books are for sale at your local
bookstore or you may call Random House at
1-800-793-BOOK to order with a credit card.*